Ethics and Governance of Public Health Information

Ethics and Governance of Public Health Information

Stephen Holland

ROWMAN &
LITTLEFIELD
INTERNATIONAL
London • New York

Published by Rowman & Littlefield International Ltd
6 Tinworth Street, London, SE11 5AL, UK
www.rowmaninternational.com

Rowman & Littlefield International Ltd.is an affiliate of Rowman & Littlefield
4501 Forbes Boulevard, Suite 200, Lanham, Maryland 20706, USA
With additional offices in Boulder, New York, Toronto (Canada), and Plymouth (UK)
www.rowman.com

British Library Cataloguing in Publication Data
A catalogue record for this book is available from the British Library

ISBN: HB 978-1-78660-055-4
PB 978-1-78660-056-1

Library of Congress Cataloging-in-Publication Data
ISBN 978-1-78660-055-4 (cloth)
ISBN 978-1-78660-056-1 (paper)
ISBN 978-1-78660-057-8 (electronic)

Contents

Dedicated with love to my parents,
Pat and Arthur Holland

Preface

This book developed out of a long-standing interest in public health ethics and research ethics. I did a book on public health ethics in 2007 (now in its second edition), looking mainly at the tensions between individual autonomy and public health, via moral and political theory. At the same time, I was setting up and running my academic department's research governance committee and later did two terms as chair of the University of York's Ethics Committee. But what really brought these themes together was the experience of setting up and chairing Public Health England's Research Governance Group (REGG). This started in 2015, and I'm very grateful to Public Health England for their initial approach and ongoing support of REGG.

Chairing REGG focused my attention on public health information, as opposed to the broader range of studies undertaken in the health sciences, or the paradigmatic clinical trial at the centre of traditional research ethics. The taxonomy of public health information presented in chapter 1 exactly mirrors the sorts and sources of information dealt with by REGG. And running REGG informed specific arguments in the book. For example, the group's initial responsibility was to ensure that research that fell outside other governance structures was properly reviewed and approved, but it quickly became obvious that it didn't make much sense to restrict the remit to research, because lots of Public Health England's research is ethically anodyne, and some standard public heath practices which generate data – surveillance, service evaluation, responses to outbreaks and so on – are ethically more contentious. Hence the extended discussion of the research–practice distinction in the first couple of chapters of this book.

But the influence goes the other way, too, because the research undertaken for this book has directly informed the work of REGG. The previous point is a good example, because the decision to review public health practices which meet certain criteria was shaped by the argument that was developing about the research–practice distinction, which ended up as chapters 1 and 2. And there is a subtler way the research for this book influenced REGG. The drift of the arguments in the book is toward a defence of public health information. Basically, I think we are in danger of prioritising privacy so much that the information required for public health is unnecessarily compromised. When we get really detailed about the sort of privacy interests or risks of harm public health information creates – and about the resources available for managing those risks, such as anonymisation, consent and trust – it turns out that we should be less anxious about public health data collection than is currently the case. This view, which developed out of the research for this book, has directly influenced the structure and mode of REGG reviews.

As I say, I'm very grateful to Public Health England for the opportunity to help devise REGG. In particular, I'd like to thank Bernie Hannigan for the initial approach and ongoing support. I've worked closely with Elizabeth Coates throughout my tenure, and I'm massively indebted to her, not just for being such a sympathetic and supportive colleague, but also for the in-depth discussions of the ethics and governance of specific public health information–gathering activities, many of which have influenced arguments in this book. Finally, I'd like to thank Rowman & Littlefield International for proposing a book on public health research ethics; in particular, Sarah Campbell, who developed the project in its early phase, and Rebecca Anastasi who took over the reins.

Introduction

Public health requires information. Traditionally, this was in the form of epidemiology, the study of the distribution and determinants of diseases in populations, but standard public health practice – such as disease surveillance and service evaluation – has always required and generated information. And public health data have recently proliferated: quantitative epidemiological methods have been augmented by diverse study designs; information gathering occurs in a range of settings, and for disparate purposes; and there is a wide and increasing variety of sorts and sources of data to inform public health.

The acquisition and use of information for public health create important issues of ethics and governance. The central problematic is a familiar trade-off between utility and privacy. On the one hand, public health information creates enormous social utility: public health is information driven, so the more data are acquired and used for public health, the better for society. But the social utility of public health information is in tension with informational privacy interests; in particular, with privacy concerns to control access to and disclosure of personal information. The ethics and governance of public health information centres on this utility-privacy dilemma.

Each chapter in this book addresses an aspect of this theme. Chapter 1 focuses the discussion by presenting a comprehensive taxonomy of public health information, categories of which include public health research, public health practice and sources of information for public health. Secondary analysis, data linkage and 'big data' are introduced and explained. The taxonomy makes the vexed distinction between research and public health practice. This raises two questions, one conceptual, the other practical. The conceptual question is whether the distinction between the concepts of research and practice can be maintained; this is addressed in chapter 1 by taking by a novel Wittgensteinian approach to defending the distinction. We should give up the hopeless search for the necessary and sufficient conditions for an activity falling under the concept of research or practice and see these as 'family resemblance concepts'.

Chapter 2 addresses the ethics and governance of public health information, which is dominated by the fault line between research and practice: all and only health related research is scrutinised, whilst public health practice escapes oversight. Given the defence of the research-practice distinction in chapter 1, this situation is conceptually respectable. But it is a form of research exceptionalism, the view that research generates particularly important risks and concerns. Strategies for defending research exceptionalism are unsuccessful. Since research exceptionalism is false, all public health information-gathering activities – research and practice – should be under the purview of ethics and governance. This appears to increase oversight beyond practicability; but research is currently overscrutinised, so proportionate review and ethical risk screening will achieve a net reduction in governance. The chapter ends with a discussion of whether – and if so, how – ethical review should be informed by public health values and goals.

Chapter 3 focuses on the value fundamental to the ethics and governance of public health information, namely, privacy. After rejecting a rights-based approach to analysing privacy, a dualistic account is presented. There are two sorts of privacy interests: to protect a private sphere in our lives, and to control personal information. This account is elucidated and defended by reference to some of the copious privacy literature. The privacy interest relevant to public health is in controlling personal information, not protecting personal space. Obscuring this distinction tends to exaggerate privacy concerns about public health data, because ambiguous talk of privacy concerns brings the weightiness of our need to protect a private sphere in our lives to bear on the discussion of public health information. In fact, privacy concerns about public health information are consequentialist: informational privacy concerns are based on the harms arising from disclosures and misuse of personal data.

Since harms are central, the first half of chapter 4 reviews literature on the concept of harm. The debate about the nature of harm is at an impasse, because numerous competing accounts are equally unsatisfactory. In response, an inclusive analysis is recommended: 'harm' will be used in the rest of the discussion to refer to any of the deleterious effects captured in the various standard accounts of harm. The second half of the chapter focuses on anonymity because, traditionally, anonymous information is considered to present no risk of harm, and whole swathes of public health data are anonymised. But traditional reliance on anonymity is challenged by reidentification science, i.e. increasingly sophisticated ways of turning anonymized into identifiable data. This challenge is met, not by querying the power of reidentification techniques, but by arguing that the risks of reidentification of public health data is already low, and can be lowered further. This argument is defended against two objections grounded in the precautionary principle and slippery slopes, respectively.

But public health cannot rely solely on anonymity, so chapter 5 discusses identifiable public health information. A novel way of trading off privacy concerns and social utility in the context of identifiable public health data is suggested: are there any pervasive influences in the way this trade-off is standardly made? It is argued that risks and harms associated with identifiable public health information are systematically overstated, in a number of subtle ways. This has the effect of weighing privacy concerns more heavily than is justified in the trade-off with social utility. The chapter also appeals to Mill's harm principle to justify identifiable public health information. The principle clearly applies in paradigm cases, such as notifiable disease reporting; it is argued that the principle can be applied further, at least to include information gathering relevantly similar to disease notification, and perhaps further still. Nonetheless, as reiterated at the end of the chapter, identifiable data can sometimes create very serious informational risks.

These informational risks need managing, and consent is a principle mechanism. But gaining consent to acquire and use public health information is often impracticable or distorts data. In response, chapter 6 distinguishes types of public health information by reference to the consent requirement. Some public health data do not raise a consent problem over and above that which arises in other contexts; other data either do not require consent, or the consent requirement is fairly easily outweighed. This distils the hard consent problem in public health down to further research uses of personal health data. The current debate about this is dominated by competing consent models and is at an impasse. So, a novel approach is recommended: consent is offset by the duty to provide one's health information for further uses. The negative part of the argument for such a duty is that objections to a general obligation to participate in medical research do not apply to health data research. The positive part is a Kantian free riding argument for a duty to contribute. The chapter ends with a discussion of how far this duty extends.

Trust is another way of managing informational risks. If public health institutions can be trusted, privacy concerns are alleviated and, in turn, restrictive data policies are unnecessary: hence the frequent calls in the literature to build trust in institutions responsible for public health data. This is fully endorsed in chapter 7. But building trust as envisaged in public health means better regulation to persuade the public that relevant institutions are reliable, and this cannot be the sole strategy. The way forward appeals to analyses of trust in other disciplines. In philosophy, trust and trustworthiness, on the one hand, are distinguished from confidence, reliance and reliability, on the other. This opens up the possibility of bolstering regulatory changes with increasing trust in, and trustworthiness of, public health institutions, as these terms are understood in philosophy. This is pursued by arguing that public health institutions are in a good position to foster public trust, because they share core values with the public. The chapter ends by illustrating how the appeal to public trust supports arguments presented in preceding chapters.

Each of the chapters just introduced can be read independently as a substantive discussion about an aspect of the ethics and governance of public health information. But there is an overarching argument which is alluded to throughout the book, fully explained in the concluding chapter and quickly sketched here. Privacy concerns are massively heightened in this 'information age'. This is understandable, but it has the inevitable effect of prioritising privacy concerns about information over its social utility. In turn, this results in restrictive data regulation and more stringent data management. But such policies tend to be generic, so they might be appropriate to some sorts of data, inappropriate to others. And public health is a case in point. The discussions in the following chapters suggest that privacy concerns and informational risks associated with public health information are overstated, and that resources for managing public health informational risks are understated. So the overall aim of this book is to defend public health information – and, in turn, public health itself – from unnecessarily restrictive data management regulation.

Chapter 1

Public Health Information and the Research-Practice Distinction

This book addresses the dilemma between social utility and personal privacy in the context of public health information, so this chapter starts by briefly describing public health. Then a complete taxonomy of public health data is presented, which will be referred to throughout the rest of the book. The categories are familiar, but the taxonomy is contentious in being based on the notoriously vexed research-practice distinction. So the second half of this chapter defends the taxonomy by addressing the conceptual problem with distinguishing research from practice. Inadequate responses to the conceptual issue are canvassed in order to get to the root of the problem. This is then addressed by presenting a Wittgensteinian solution: 'research' and 'practice' are family resemblance concepts, which we understand and deploy despite there being no defining set of necessary or sufficient conditions of either. In turn, there is no conceptual objection to a taxonomy that makes the research-practice distinction.

PUBLIC HEALTH

A good way to conceptualise public health is by contrast with clinical medicine. Clinical medicine is concerned with the diagnosis and treatment of individual patients in institutional health care contexts. Typically, an individual presents at a primary care facility with symptoms; a primary care doctor then diagnoses and treats the patient, or refers him or her to secondary and tertiary level providers. By contrast, the focus of public health is not the individual patient but populations of people; hence the phrases 'population health' to refer to public health and 'population perspective' to capture the public health standpoint. Populations are of different sizes and compositions, from subsections of a country's citizenry to entire nation-states and even – as captured by 'global health' – the entire world. But whatever the population in question, the dual aim of public health is the same: to protect and promote the health of populations and to reduce health inequalities within populations.

There is a second important defining characteristic of public health. The aims of public health can be achieved only by collective state-backed action. This is a two-fold necessary condition on effective public health. Collective action is required because public health interventions work only if all members of the population in question – or, at least, a sufficiently large proportion of them – are prepared to contribute to public health endeavours. So the benefits of public health are communal, and require communal activity. And public health requires state support, since public health initiatives are instigated, devised, implemented, evaluated and sanctioned by instruments of the state, in the form of government funded public health institutions. Typically, these include public health observatories and laboratories, and a network of state-funded public health bodies and professionals. In sum, public health comprises collective state-backed action to protect and promote the health of populations, and to reduce health inequalities within populations.

Illustrations of public health interventions can be usefully divided into those aiming to prevent ill-health and those aiming to promote better health. Examples of the former include vaccination or mass immunization campaigns, the aim of which is to prevent the spread of disease; screening programmes are designed to detect conditions in asymptomatic populations which respond to early treatment; and public health responses to emergencies or outbreak situations are intended to ameliorate the threat of a sudden population health risk. By contrast, health promotion activities aim to improve, as opposed to merely protect, health status. These centre on individuals' health related behaviour, and include providing information about healthy lifestyle choices, and motivating behaviour change to improve current health levels, whilst making people less susceptible to ill health. Familiar examples include campaigns to get people to quit smoking, eat healthily and take more exercise.

TAXONOMY OF PUBLIC HEALTH DATA

The acquisition and use of health related information is vital to all the aspects of public health just sketched. The following is intended as an exhaustive categorisation of public health information-gathering activities. The taxonomy has three main categories: public health research; public health practice; and sources of information which can be accessed for public health purposes. The taxonomy ends with a comment on how these forms of public health information gathering relate to the traditional science of public health, namely, epidemiology.

Public Health Research

The standard definition of research is, 'a systematic investigation, including research development, testing, and evaluation, designed to develop or contribute to generalizable knowledge' (Code of Federal Regulations). This definition, taken from the 'Common Rule' – i.e., the US Federal Policy for the Protection of Human Subjects – has two parts. 'Systematic investigation' means an activity that is planned in advance, and which collects and uses data to answer a question or meet a research objective. 'Generalizable knowledge' refers to information that fills a knowledge gap or expands the knowledge base of the field of study in question, as opposed to being applicable only to the context in which it is collected. Typically, research involves testing a hypothesis using proven research methods – as alluded to in the Common Rule – such as controlled trials and experimental techniques: in sum, the scientific method as applied in the field of public health.

Public Health Practice: Surveillance, Data Collection During Emergencies and Service Evaluation

Public health practice includes three main activities which involve information gathering: surveillance; data collection in response to emergencies or outbreaks; and service evaluation. To take each in turn, public health surveillance systems monitor the health of populations and are standardly defined as 'ongoing, systematic collection, analysis and interpretation of health-related data essential to the planning, implementation, and evaluation of public health practice' (WHO). There are two important parts to this definition. First, information is routinely acquired in an ongoing and systematic fashion, as opposed to occasional or episodic data collection. Second, surveillance data are collected in order to inform public health activities; as the WHO definition goes on to say, surveillance can 'serve as an early warning system for major public health threats and disease outbreaks; document the impact of an intervention, or track progress towards specified goals; and monitor and clarify the epidemiology of health problems, to allow priorities to be set and to inform public health policy and strategies'.

This simplistic definition of surveillance is deceptive and masks a number of complications. For one thing, since surveillance systems are designed to monitor specific conditions, they differ markedly from one another, especially between health care settings which vary in terms of how well developed the health system is, how sophisticated are the available data collection methods, the socio-political acceptability of different sorts of monitoring, and the kinds of public health threats which exist (Nsubugu et al. 2006: 1006-1015; WHO 2017: 14–16). Surveillance might be defined more or less broadly. A broad definition will encompass any continuing scrutiny which pertains to disease control, including, for example, non-health specific information such as registering births and deaths, and epidemiological research. The sort and amount of surveillance data varies, from handwritten paper records to sophisticated electronic and digital data, and can include information on communicable and non-communicable diseases, registers of notifiable diseases, accidents and injuries, recording health care activities, and so on. Notwithstanding these disparities, the 'Common Rule' definition captures the basic features of all surveillance systems, which indicate that surveillance is a distinctive way of 'knowing about health' (Lee and Thacker 2011).

As suggested by the WHO quote above, a major objective of surveillance is to alert public health authorities to 'major public health threats and disease outbreaks'. This introduces the second sort of public health practice, namely, data collection during public emergencies. Outbreaks of infectious diseases are central public health emergencies, including well publicised cases such as SARS (Severe Acute Respiratory Syndrome), FHF (Filovirus Haemorrhagic Fevers, notably Marburg and Ebola), and the Zika virus. Such infectious diseases are characterised by the speed and rapidity with which epidemics can spread, including across national borders, necessitating a quick and internationally concerted response. But 'emergencies' also covers less standard cases. For example, antimicrobial resistance (AMR) – where microorganisms develop such that antibiotics, antivirals and antimalarials stop working so standard treatments become ineffective – has been described as a 'slowly emerging public health disaster' (Viens and Littmann 2015). Along another dimension, humanitarian crises which are not solely or specifically health emergencies can have serious public health consequences. This includes conflict and terror-related emergencies, mass migrations of people, and extreme weather events (Mitra and Sethi 2016).

In a well-used phrase, WHO states: 'During an infectious disease outbreak there is a moral obligation to learn as much as possible as quickly as possible, in order to inform the ongoing public health response, and to allow for proper scientific evaluation of new interventions being tested.' Learning 'as much as possible' in emergency contexts is multifaceted, ranging from identifying the causes and risk factors of disease, and determining the extent of an outbreak, to recommending and evaluating health programmatic responses. Relevant techniques for acquiring information include rapid needs assessment, and population surveys to determine current health status and assess programme coverage (Johnson and Vindrola-Padros 2017). As the WHO quote indicates, given the seriousness and speed with which such public health emergencies develop, information gathering in such situations typically necessitates quickly constructing and implementing a method for collecting data.

A third sort of public health practice is service evaluation. This is grounded in public health's remit to ensure the provision and quality of, and access to, health services. Service evaluation is ambiguous between two sorts of seemingly similar activities which take different perspectives on existing services. One sort of service evaluation, usually referred to as quality assurance or audit, is intended to review how care is being delivered; in particular, to ensure that the service in question is being provided to 'a predetermined standard' (Chen and Fawcett 2017: 3). The second sort of service evaluation, usually referred to as quality improvement, involves designing, implementing and testing innovations in existing services in order to improve them. Although distinguishable, the aims of both sorts of evaluation are the same – to ensure good service provision – and the two are often related, for example when an audit reveals problems with a service which motivates a quality improvement activity (Grembowski 2015).

Service evaluation is a traditional feature of public health, but recent developments are increasingly influencing the field. One now quite well established variant is 'patient safety research' which starts the evaluative process by studying adverse events in medical and health care settings, with a view to identifying and understanding poor service provision (Mannion and Braithwaite 2017). Another is the burgeoning 'learning health care system' approach, defined by the Institute of Medicine as 'one in which knowledge generation is so embedded into the core of the practice of medicine that it is a natural outgrowth and product of the healthcare delivery process and leads to continual improvement in care' (Olsen, Aisner and McGinnis 2007: 6). Advocates see learning health care systems as the most effective way of achieving the goals of traditional quality improvement, and appeal to health care institutions to systematically acquire transparent evidence of the quality of care being provided (Faden et al. 2013).

Three Sources of Information for Public Health: Health Activity Data, Biobanks and Novel Forms of Health Information

A striking characteristic of the health sector is that an enormous amount of health activity information is collected at all points of health care provision. Although this varies between health care contexts depending on contingent factors – whether local means for data collection and storage are well developed, for example – all health care systems at least attempt to document activity, because this is universally important in managing the treatment of individual patients (Fritz, Tilahun and Dugas 2015). Two well-known features of the English health care system are illustrative. At the primary level, the medical history of all NHS patients have been recorded since the inception of the service in order to facilitate treatment management. The main innovation here is the shift from paper-based records and charts to electronic health records (EHR) – also referred to as electronic medical records (EMR) – made possible by developments in information technology (Pagliari, Detmer and Singleton 2007). And at the secondary and tertiary levels, hospital activity is recorded in Hospital Episode Statistics (HES), a database that details admissions, attendances at Accident and Emergency Departments, and outpatient appointments for NHS hospitals in England (NHS Digital).

An example of how such information is useful to public health – and which illustrates recent trends in data management – is the English NHS 'national data opt-out programme' (NHS Digital[a]). The programme was introduced in May 2018 and replaces the 'types 1 and 2' opt-outs that were put in place in 2014 (NHS Digital[b]). The new programme is designed to make it easier for patients to opt-out of their confidential information being used for purposes of research and planning, including the facility to directly set one's opt-out preferences online (or using convenient off-line alternatives). In an insightful comment, Piel et al. (2018) endorse the right to opt-out, but sound a number of cautionary notes, on behalf of public health. Generally, 'prevalence of opt-outs has been slowly increasing over time between April 2016 and December 2017' (p. 3). More specifically, Piel et al. show that the distribution of opt-outs is nonrandom, because they are influenced by demographic factors. In turn, this introduces biases that have 'important implications for the generalizability of public health research' (p. 3), citing in particular the effects on surveillance and environmental health projects.

A second source of information for public health is biobanks. Collection and storage of human specimens has a century-long history, but the main developments in biobanking have occurred in the past two or three decades, largely due to technological advances and increased capacity to harvest and store biological materials from routine medical interventions (De Souza and Greenspan 2013: 304–5). As Brand, Schulte and Probst-Hensch (2012: 6) point out, the 'definition of biobanking is very wide', resulting in pleas for what Fransson et al. (2015) call a 'common language of biobanking.' Nonetheless, and as Brand, Schulte, and Probst-Hensch go on to suggest, biobanking at its most basic 'has a twofold character comprising both samples and data…[Biobanks] can be defined as collections of samples of human body substances (e.g. cells, tissue, blood or DNA) that are or can be associated with individual data and information such as clinical, socioeconomic, demographic, lifestyle, behavioural and environmental health determinants' (p. 6–7).

The current situation regarding biobanks is complex. There are various sorts of biorepositories; Paskal et al. (2018: 772), for example, distinguish 'population-based, disease-oriented, and tissue biobanks'. In the background here is a broader distinction between therapeutic biobanks aimed at personalised medicine versus large-scale population-based biobanks (Burke et al. 2010). A number of types of biobanks have been established across the globe (De Souza and Greenspan 2013: Table 1; Paskal et al. 2018: Table 1); although these all accept, process, store and distribute biospecimens and associated data for use in research and clinical care, their management and governance vary markedly among sociocultural settings. This ushers in international guidelines for best practice in designing and operating biobanks, notably by the International Society for Biological and Environmental Repositories (ISBER; see Campbell et al. 2018).

The future of biobanking is somewhat unclear. Chalmers et al. (2016) sound a sceptical note, pointing out the lack of convergence on a model for biobanking and the failure of biobanks to achieve long-term sustainability. In particular, they predict 'that the vastly expensive population-wide biobank model is unlikely to survive in its current form for much longer' (p. 11). More optimistic prospects for biobanks include developing biobanking ontology (in the computer science sense) to link with '-omics data' to integrate information from diverse biobanks (Brochhausen et al. 2016).

The third source of public health information is a direct product of the 'digital age'. The use of the Internet, social media, and online sharing platforms is now very widespread and seems set to increase in terms of technological sophistication and geographical coverage. These create novel online sources of public health data which can be categorised in various ways (Vayena, Mastroianni and Kahn 2012). Some information is explicitly health related, but much is not, including general Internet activity, social network postings and online consumer trends (Paul and Dredze 2017). Although information is initially provided voluntarily, data mining of large data sets generates further information without the knowledge of individuals. These novel online sources of information are or could be used to support all aspects of public health research and practice, including surveillance and monitoring – such as early (real-time) detection of disease outbreaks – and for longer-term public health purposes; for example, detecting patterns in health behaviour and attitudes, and pharmacovigilance.

Some specific examples will illustrate the phenomenon. The 'Patients LikeMe' network enables patients with the same condition to share experiences and thereby generate data about their disease. Web facilities such as Google Trends and Google Insights for Search analyse aggregate Internet search behaviour, which can in turn reveal health trends. There is burgeoning literature on the use of social media data for public health purposes: Twitter in particular (Sinnenberg et al. 2017), but also other social media platforms, such as Instagram (Muralidhara and Paul 2018) and Facebook (Gittelman et al. 2015). A related but distinctive phenomenon is crowdsourcing for public health. Although its definition is disputed, crowdsourcing is characterised by large groups of people collectively solving a problem or completing a task, specifically by soliciting and combining Web-based contributions. Wazny (2018) documents crowdsourcing for public health purposes, notably for surveillance during public health emergencies (see also Créquit at al. 2018). A related feature is digital storytelling, a form of participatory research in which individuals use widely available media production techniques (such as digital cameras and voice recorders) to create short narratives that can be shared online or via other electronic distribution systems (Tsui and Stareheski 2018).

Cross-Cutting Themes: Secondary Analysis, Data Linkage and 'Big Data'

Three current features of information and information technology cross-cut the categories distinguished here. 'Secondary analysis' refers to further uses of data for purposes other than that for which it was originally collected; so the challenging aspect of any sort of secondary data analysis is the permissibility of using someone's information for purposes other than that to which they originally consented. 'Data linkage' is made possible by powerful information technology systems which allow information from different data sets to be brought together in an unprecedented fashion. Two aspects of data linkage are notable: linked information is about the same individual or entity (such as place or event), and data linkage creates new data sets that are richer than the originals. 'Big data' refers not just to the size of a data set – typically, too big to be managed by traditional data-processing software – but to what has become known as 'the three Vs': variety, volume and velocity (two other Vs are sometimes added, value and veracity, further indicating that big data is characterized less by size than by what can be done with it).

These features of information technology are increasingly well established and currently under extensive discussion in public health. Secondary analyses are common in public health: data from all three sources of information for public health delineated here – health activity data, biobanks and online resources – can be used further to the original purpose; and secondary analysis can enhance both research and public health practice (Boslaugh 2007). Linkage of data sets is also prevalent, including data sets collected for research and other purposes, such as information from electronic patient records, cancer registries and socioeconomic surveys (Wellcome Trust 2015). And the promise of big data in public health has been said to include 'providing insights into the causes and outcomes of disease, better drug targets . . . enhanced disease prediction and prevention . . . improve our understanding of health behaviors (smoking, drinking, etc.)' (Khoury and Ioannidis 2014; see also Lane et al. 2014). Of course, these three features of information technology for public health are interconnected: linking data sets is a form of secondary analysis, data linkage creates big data, and so on.

A final comment before critiquing this taxonomy: how do these categories of information for public health relate to epidemiology, the traditional term for the 'science of public health' which undertakes quantitative analysis of the incidence, distribution, and possible control of diseases, illnesses and other factors? Nothing hangs on verbal issues, but it is worth noting that the term 'epidemiology' is avoided here in order to avoid a distorting reduction of the complexities of public health information to a single subject. It seems more sensible to stipulate expansively and think of all categories of public health information described here as aspects of epidemiology. Public health research, practice, and novel sources of information are all in the service of improved public health, which is the point of epidemiology; but a convincing analysis requires maintaining the distinctions between sorts of information for public health made in the taxonomy (cf. CIOMS 2009: 14).

THE RESEARCH–PRACTICE DISTINCTION

The taxonomy presented in the previous section is contentious in making the distinction between research and public health practice, which is notoriously fraught. Comments such as 'the research-practice distinction cannot be maintained' are very common. But such comments are ambiguous. The claim could be conceptual, i.e. 'research' and 'practice' seem to mean or refer to different things when in fact they do not. Or the claim could be practical: even if we can, conceptually speaking, distinguish research from practice, we should not do so for governance purposes. These two claims need to be considered separately, so the conceptual issue is dealt with in this chapter, and the practical question is addressed in the next chapter. The position defended in these discussions is that the research–practice distinction can be maintained on conceptual grounds, but the ethics and governance of public health information should not be based on the distinction.

The Conceptual Problem

The conceptual objection to the research–practice distinction is straightforward: there is no defining characteristic of all and only research. In other words, whenever a definition is presented which identifies features of research, it turns out that not all research activities, and some nonresearch activities, exhibit those features; so the putative definition fails to demarcate research as a type of activity distinct from public health practice. Incidentally, this issue is not confined to public health: 'Drawing a sharp distinction between research and therapy can be appealing [but activities] cannot be comfortably classified as either research or therapy' (Kass et al. 2013: S4), a variant on the problem which is particularly pressing in the context of the 'learning health care system' (see also Beauchamp and Saghai 2012: 49).

The problem can be illustrated by the standard definition of research taken from the 'Common Rule' presented above: 'a systematic investigation . . . designed to develop or contribute to generalizable knowledge'. As Otto, Holodniy and DeFraites (2014: 596) put it,

> attempts to differentiate research from public health practice . . . through the rubrics of the Common Rule are problematic in light of their overlapping spheres . . . 'systematic investigations' producing 'generalizable knowledge' can describe . . . public health activities – such as surveillance, emergency response, and program evaluation – as well as human participant research.

The point is well established in relevant literature, but an interesting question not often addressed is whether the two components in the Common Rule definition – 'systematic investigation' and 'generalizable knowledge' – are equally bad at singling out research.

The obvious thought is that 'systematic investigation' is really hopeless, because surely all public health practice is investigative and systematic. An unsystematic population health surveillance system is oxymoronic, and how could a rapid investigation of a disease outbreak be anything other than investigative? Related to this is the frequently mentioned fact that research and practice share data collection methods, in that both these sets of activities employ standard quantitative (controlled trials, survey questionnaires, etc.) and qualitative methodologies (thematic analysis of focus group discussions, semistructured interviews, etc.). By contrast, a defence of the research-practice distinction on grounds of 'generalizable knowledge' seems stronger, because public health practice activities address discrete informational goals – acquiring data on the prevalence of a particular condition in a particular population, the extent of a specific disease outbreak, or the quality of a given service, for example – by which their findings are restricted; whereas, by contrast, research generates knowledge that is more generally applicable.

But though it might not seem so obvious, generalizability alone is just as bad at singling out research. The very notion of generalizability is problematic because all information is somewhat generalizable and no information is entirely generalizable. As Hodge (2005: 127) pointed out, it is particularly inapt to 'public health activities that, by their nature, focus on populations rather than individuals.' The point applies to both research and practice. Regarding the former, lots of research objectives are specific and contained; and no matter how widely applicable the results, they are restricted at least to the subject matter or field of enquiry in question. Even the results of a clinical trial – a paradigmatic research study – are generalizable only to the drug or health technology under investigation. Conversely, information generated by public health practice is always to some extent generalizable. For example, results from a service audit – a putative paradigm of nonresearch – can be used to infer the quality of an equivalent service elsewhere or in the future. And some public health practice explicitly aims at generalizable information; the difference between passive and sentinel surveillance systems, for instance, is that the latter is conducted only in certain selected sites, the findings being extrapolated to the population being monitored.

Responses to the Problem

One response is to suggest defining characteristics of research other than those in the Common Rule. This is a prominent strategy in the literature, but a couple of illustrations show how unpromising it is. A well-established suggestion is that the defining characteristic of research is the intention or purpose for which it is undertaken: 'The major distinction between research and practice is in the intent for which the activity was designed' (Snider and Stroup 1997: 32; see also Gostin and Hodge 2004: 9; Otto, Holodniy, and DeFraites 2014: 596). But often this move just collapses back into the Common Rule definition – for example, Snider and Stroup (1997: 32) immediately go on to say: 'The intent of research is to contribute to or generate generalizable knowledge' – and this has already been found wanting. To work, the appeal to intentions would have to make the substantive claim that research and practice are undertaken with different intent; but a widely acknowledged fundamental reason that it is hard to distinguish research and practice is precisely that they have the same goals: 'Both [primary care] research and [public health] surveillance involve collection and analysis of individual health information to improve the health of individuals, communities, and populations' (Lussier et al. 2012: 117).

Another suggestion is to base the research–practice distinction on the different benefits they accrue, respectively. For example, one of the ways the Centers for Disease Control and Prevention (CDC) distinguished research and nonresearch is that the 'intended benefits' of the former 'can include study participants, but always extend beyond the study participants, usually to society' whilst the 'intended benefits' of the latter 'are primarily or exclusively for the participants (or clients) or the participants' community' (CDC 2010: 3; see also Snider and Stroup 1997: 30; Gostin and Hodge 2004: 9; Hodge 2005: 127). Again, this could just be an iteration of the generalizability criterion – i.e. research is generalizable in the sense that it benefits society in general – in which case it does not add to the unsatisfactory Common Rule definition. And to the extent that it is a substantive claim, it is clearly hopeless. The benefits promised by research projects can be more or less extensively distributed – a randomised control trial of a drug to treat a rare condition does not promise benefits 'to the whole of society' – and conversely, the benefits of public health practice almost always extend widely (a surveillance system benefits the entire population, for example). Hence the odd attempt by the CDC to draw a distinction based on benefitting 'society' versus 'community', as though these are different things.

We could go on, but the point is clear: putative defining characteristics of research either collapse back into the Common Rule definition or are unconvincing. Evidently, defining research and distinguishing it from public health practice remain vexed so a taxonomy of public health information which trades on the distinction, such as the one presented in the first half of this chapter, is conceptually dubious. But there is an unfamiliar way through this familiar impasse.

Beyond Definitions

To introduce this, consider some further details in the literature on the research–practice distinction. First, question-begging – i.e. assuming in an argument that which is in question – is persistent. In this case, the question is begged when arguments for the research–practice distinction assume the research–practice distinction. This happens, for example, when the distinction is based on differences in the way these activities are treated. A case in point is Gostin and Hodge (2004: 50), who suggest that 'general legal authorization supports a finding of public health practice': this assumes that there is a practice–research distinction for legal bodies to make when authorizing activities, which is precisely what is in question. Closely connected to this is the tendency in the literature to provide circular definitions. In fact, this started with the Common Rule, which defined research in terms of '*research* development, testing, and evaluation': research is defined in terms of research development and, presumably, vice versa. An egregious example is: 'Any intent to conduct research supports a finding that the activity, at least in part, is research' (Gostin and Hodge 2004: 9).

Question-begging arguments and circular definitions suggest a way out of the impasse regarding the research–practice distinction that is hinted at by Fairchild and Bayer (2004: 632): 'recent efforts to provide definitional solutions to the question of research and public health practice involve twists and turns that inevitably produce results that are riddled with inconsistencies and that are conceptually unsatisfying'. As this indicates, the root of the problem is the insistence on giving definitions to maintain distinctions; i.e. on defining research, as opposed to public health practice, or on proffering defining characteristics of one or other of these activities (traditionally by providing necessary and sufficient conditions for an activity being research or practice). This creates the quandary. An object of conceptual analysis – in this case, an information-gathering activity, namely, research or public health practice – is distinguished by a putative definition; for example, research is defined in terms of aiming at generalizable knowledge, as in the Common Rule. This is queried by dint of counter-examples; i.e. research that lacks the putative defining characteristic or nonresearch practices that have it (for example, research which does not produce generalizable findings or public health practice which does). Reiterate the pattern often enough – replace generalizable knowledge with intent, benefit, etc., as illustrated above – and the inevitable result is scepticism that the objects of analysis can be defined and distinguished at all (in this case, that we can define research and thereby distinguish it from practice).

The solution is to root out the problem by eschewing 'definitional solutions to the question of research and public health practice.' To begin, note that we already grasp the difference between research and public health practice. We must do; otherwise, we could not undertake the process of refuting putative definitions by counter-examples. To recall the illustrations already mentioned, how could we say that generalizability – or intent, benefit or whatever – is not a defining characteristic of research unless we already have a pretty good grasp of what research is? Likewise, this explains the question-begging and circularity: writers assume the research–practice distinction in their arguments for it, or define research in terms of research, because we already have an understanding of it. So it appears that we know what these activities are and how they differ from one another, yet we cannot settle on defining characteristics (or necessary and sufficient conditions) of them. This seems paradoxical. But there is a quite different approach to the issue which deploys well-established philosophical resources other than 'definitional solutions' to dispel the air of paradox.

A Wittgensteinian Defence of the Research–Practice Distinction

This approach is, broadly speaking, Wittgensteinian, since it draws on Wittgenstein's (2009) later writings. The basic idea is that we can grasp a concept, activity, practice or institution despite the fact that we struggle to provide a satisfying definition. This seems to be exactly what we need to get through the research–practice impasse. A few details will be enough to develop the idea for present purposes. At the heart of the approach is anti-essentialism, i.e. the view that there is no essence of the thing in question (in this case, research). This is why putative definitions fail: definitions are supposed to capture the essence of the definiendum – traditionally, by providing necessary and sufficient conditions – so they are bound to disappoint if there is no essence to capture. How, then, do we understand, recognise or know about the thing in question, in this case research? A quick way into the Wittgensteinian response is his notion of 'family resemblance concepts' (Wennerberg 1967).

Literally speaking, members of a family sometimes share a 'family resemblance'; there is no one thing they all have in common – exactly the same length of nose, or whatever – but they share an overlapping series of similarities by which others recognise them to be related. Analogously, 'family resemblance concepts' pick out things which are not connected by any one essential or common feature, but which share a series of similarities. Wittgenstein's famous illustration of a 'family resemblance concept' is 'games'. We understand, recognise, know about games, yet, on reflection, we can see that there is no one thing all games have in common, no essential feature of games. Hence, there is no satisfying definition of 'game'. Rather, games have a 'family resemblance' in that they share in 'a complicated network of similarities overlapping and criss-crossing' (Wittgenstein 2009: 66).

Wittgenstein's remarks on family resemblance are part of a larger approach to language and meaning which were his primary concerns – as opposed to conceptual analysis of 'game' or whatever – and which includes other famous Wittgensteinian notions such as 'language games', 'forms of life' and 'rule-following'. We do not need to go further into these for present purposes; the basic idea is to think of research activities and public health practice as family resemblance concepts. This is a familiar move in myriad disparate debates; for example, McKinnon (2002) and Haugaard (2010) take this approach to the problem of defining religion and power, respectively. Applying this to the research–practice distinction is to embrace the fact that there is no one essential feature common to all and only research activities. This is why definitions of research fail. Yet we recognise research activities as distinct from other activities. This is because they share a 'network of similarities'. When we argue for the research–practice distinction, we end up begging the question, and when we proffer definitions they end up being circular, because we already recognise research activities by the family resemblance they share.

Some commentators have come close to this Wittgensteinian way of addressing the conceptual problem in distinguishing research and practice. For example, Goldberg (2011) offers precisely a 'family resemblance analysis', but his focus is on the therapeutic misconception as opposed to the research–practice distinction. On the other hand, Bortolotti and Heinrichs (2007) attempt to define, delimit and demarcate research. Their analysis has much in common with the Wittgensteinian approach taken here. In particular, they are imaginatively inclusive about the dimensions of research – they include functional and procedural dimensions, for example – and accept that 'research shares certain features with other human activities', as opposed to insisting that research is 'delimited' by a unique feature. But nonetheless, Bortolotti and Heinrichs are still in the business of providing a definition 'which tells us whether an activity is research' (Holm 2007: 154; see also Bortolotti and Heinrichs's Table 1, p. 168). This inevitably results in a questionable reductionism of the sort avoided by the Wittgensteinian approach recommended here.

Challenges

Two sorts of objections to the analysis presented here centre on the requisite 'networks of similarities' shared by research and practice, respectively. On the one hand, it could be that research and practice share a family resemblance with one another, as opposed to these being two distinct activities which bear only internal resemblance. For example, as Otto, Holodniy and DeFraites (2014: 597) point out, there are 'elements common to public health practice and research.' But this objection confuses the fact that research and practice have some things in common with family resemblance, which is based on 'a complicated network of similarities overlapping and criss-crossing.' Individual, discrete elements can be shared by concepts or activities which we already understand to be distinct from one another. So, for example, 'games' and 'politics' have some 'common elements' – both are competitive, for example – but no one infers from this that they are indistinguishable; likewise, research and practice.

On the other hand, it could be objected that various research activities do not have enough in common to create a family resemblance. For example, two research studies might seem wildly divergent in terms of aims, design, methods, participants and so on. But this objection is a case in point of continuing to think in terms of defining characteristics of these activities. There are lots of lists of features of research and practice, respectively, in the literature; a nice illustration is Gostin and Hodge's (2004) discussion of numerous criteria for distinguishing research and practice. But because they are continuing the quest for 'essential characteristics of public health practice or research' (p. 48), Gostin and Hodge consider each criterion as a defining characteristic of research or practice, and either reject or endorse it as such. By contrast, on the approach recommended here, these are not lists of putative defining characteristics of one or another activity; rather, they are similarities shared by each of these activities, respectively, which create the family resemblance between research activities, on the one hand, and the family resemblance between public health practices on the other.

Family resemblance concepts are closely connected to vague concepts (Biletzki and Matar 2018). 'Vague' in philosophy does not mean imprecise or unclear. Rather, a philosophically vague concept or predicate is one that admits of borderline cases in which there is no fact of the matter – no right answer – as to whether it applies. 'Tall' is vague in this sense. Some people are tall, some not tall, but there is no 'bright line' between tall and not tall people, no cut off point at which people go from being not tall to tall. The literature on the research–practice distinction is awash with references to research and practice as vague concepts, often in terms of a grey area between the two: there is a 'gray borderland' (Fairchild and Bayer 2004: 632), 'all shades of grey' (Wade 2005), a 'gray zone' (Hodge 2005: 125) between them. But it is a mistake to infer from a grey area anything deeply problematic about the research–practice distinction.

Note first that vague boundaries are still boundaries. Some people are tall, others not tall, despite 'tall' being a vague concept. Likewise, even if research is a vague concept, it 'will be possible to describe some activities as pure research and some other activities as pure practice' (Levine 1975: 1). So it would not follow from vagueness that distinctions between research and practice are 'artificial' (Willison et al. 2014); certainly not that they are 'arbitrary' or these activities 'cannot be distinguished in a reliable or valid way' (Wade 2005).

Of course, if any putative 'gray zone' between research and practice is massive, we are left with a practical – as opposed to conceptual – problem. And this is often implied in the literature: 'Lost in a . . . gray zone are a host of public health activities' (Hodge 2005: 125); 'Most everyone in public health knows how difficult it can be to distinguish between practice and research beyond the easiest of cases' (Gostin and Hodge 2004: 7). But this seems precisely the wrong round: the vast majority of activities are easy cases in terms of recognising whether they are research or practice, because we understand these concepts and grasp their deployment, so any 'grey zone' would consist of only a small minority of hard cases on the borderline between two vague concepts.

One thing that creates the false impression that the 'grey zone' between research and practice is sizeable is that writers often confuse complications around the research–practice distinction with vagueness. For example, an activity might start out as nonresearch but segue into a research activity; alternatively, a project might include both research and practice components (CDC 2010). Both of these might seem to sit in a grey area between research and practice but, in fact, neither entails vagueness. The former describes two phases of a project at different times, in the first of which it is public health practice, in the second it is a research study. The latter describes a study which is complex in that it includes research and practice components which, at least in principle, can be disentangled.

CONCLUDING REMARKS

This chapter focused the discussion on public health as a domain of information. A taxonomy of public health information was presented; this makes the notorious research–practice distinction, so the conceptual question as to whether we can maintain this distinction in light of persistent failures of putative definitions was addressed. The suggestion is that we can, by replacing definitional solutions to the question of research and public health practice with a Wittgensteinian approach that sees research and practice as family resemblance concepts. In turn, the taxonomy presented here, which makes the research–practice distinction, is conceptually sound. But the next question is practical: should the research–practice distinction inform the ethics and governance of these activities to the extent to which it currently does? This is addressed in the next chapter.

Chapter 2

Governance, Research Exceptionalism and Proportionate Review

This chapter turns from conceptual to practical matters raised by public health information. In current regulatory systems, all and only research requires ethical review and formal approval by ethics committees. To refer back to the taxonomy of public health data presented in the previous chapter, all and only public health research has ethical and governance oversight. Given the defence of the research–practice distinction in the previous chapter, this is conceptually tenable. But it is highly questionable: is it necessary to scrutinise all research studies; should nonresearch activities which generate data undergo ethical review?

The argument of this chapter is as follows. The current regulatory system is a form of research exceptionalism, i.e. all and only research requires scrutiny, because it is exceptionally risky. Two strategies for defending research exceptionalism are discussed; both fail, so research exceptionalism is shown to be false. In turn, the current system of scrutinising all and only research is ethically untenable. But this creates a serious practical problem. Unless oversight is restricted to research, there will be a massive increase in the number of projects which require ethics review and approval. This sort of governance inflation is highly undesirable, so the second half of this chapter argues that increased regulation of public health information can be avoided by invoking proportionate review and better ethical risk screening. The upshot is that we can bring all public health information under the purview of ethics and governance without massively inflating ethical oversight and governance. The chapter ends with a discussion of the sort of review appropriate to public health data.

RESEARCH EXCEPTIONALISM

Ethical review typically involves objective, independent, third-party scrutiny of projects by ethics committees, such as Research Ethics Committees (RECs) and Independent Review Boards (IRBs) in the UK and US, respectively. Ethical review is required for all and only research studies; conversely, nonresearch activities do not require ethics committee approval. As Hansson (2011: 22) puts it, 'the boundary between research and non-research will often determine the ethical demands on an activity, so that the demands on it are higher if it falls on the research side of the boundary.' This boundary between research and nonresearch is drawn in public health information in particular. To recall the public health information taxonomy from the previous chapter, there is ethical oversight of all research undertaken to support public health, including ethical scrutiny and stringent regulation, but not of public health practices which generate information for public health.

Many commentators object to this established regulatory system of ethical oversight of all and only research on the conceptual grounds that the distinction between research and public health practice cannot be maintained. Given the defence of the research–practice distinction in the last chapter, this move is clearly unavailable here. In other words, in light of the previous chapter, there is no conceptual objection to scrutinising all and only research. Of course, there will be some contestable cases in the 'grey area' between research and practice, as discussed in the previous chapter, but no deep conceptual objection to the current governance system. But whilst there is no conceptual problem with scrutinising all and only research, it is ethically highly questionable.

The current regulatory system of stringently regulating all and only research is a form of 'research exceptionalism', i.e. the view that research is distinct from nonresearch activities in a way that grounds particularly close scrutiny. So we can address the current regulatory framework by asking whether research exceptionalism is justified. The key is to distinguish two strategies by which research exceptionalism might be defended. The first strategy is to justify research exceptionalism on the grounds that research is riskier than other activities; the second is to accept that research is no riskier than other activities, but provides other grounds for stringent regulation. The argument here is that both strategies fail, so research exceptionalism is unjustified.

Risk of Harm as Grounds for Research Exceptionalism

The first strategy is that research exceptionalism is justified because research is distinctive in creating serious risks of harm, so it requires particularly close scrutiny and stricter regulation. This is a common interpretation of research exceptionalism in the literature, as the 'practice of treating research risks with greater caution than we treat other risks' (Rivera 2014: 49). The strategy is exemplified by Hansson (2011: 24–26), who discusses four 'possible justifications for the practice of placing higher ethical demands on an activity when it is part of research than otherwise', the first of which is, 'research is more dangerous or has worse effects'.

Initially, this strategy seems hopeless. As is frequently pointed out in the literature, there are innumerable counter-examples to the claim that research is especially risky. For example, Wilson and Hunter (2010: 48) describe 'activities which are clearly not research, but which nonetheless impose similar or greater risks than much research, but which are typically not nearly so stringently regulated'. They cite four from 'any number of such examples', namely, journalism, reality TV shows, dangerous sports and government action. As this list indicates, the point applies both to nonresearch activities which do not involve gathering information – sports, for example – and those that do, such as journalism.

Add to this that some research activities create no or only minimal risk, and it seems obvious that research is not a type of activity that is exceptional compared to others in being risky, so this first strategy for defending research exceptionalism fails. But it can be pursued a little further. The premise that 'research is riskier than other activities' is ambiguous between creating risk *per se* and creating idiosyncratic sorts of risks. Take the premise in the former way and it is quickly dismissed, because it is easy to find counter-examples of research that does not, and nonresearch activity that does, create risks. But that leaves the second reading. Perhaps it is not risk *per se*, but idiosyncratic sorts of risk that justify research exceptionalism.

For example, Wilson and Hunter (2010: 49–50) discuss risk *per se*, but go on to present three further risk-related features of research: noncomprehended risk (due to the incomprehensibility of research protocols); risk of undue inducement (primarily by being paid to participate); and risk of exploitation (i.e. entering into an unfair bargain between researchers and participants). Such risk-related features of research seem idiosyncratic, so might be taken as a defence of research exceptionalism. But Wilson and Hunter themselves do an excellent job of showing that these are 'unsuccessful arguments' (p. 49), because such features are not really idiosyncratic to research; rather, they are common in other walks of life – which we do not and should not stringently regulate – so they do not justify research exceptionalism.

There is one final thing to say about this first, risk-based strategy for defending research exceptionalism. It seems odd that research came to be seen as riskier than other activities, when it so clearly is not. But there is a standard explanation for this. Thinking of research as particularly risky is an overreaction to what Wilson and Hunter (2010: 49) rather drily refer to as 'something of a checkered past', i.e. well-documented and widely publicised historical research scandals. These include notorious atrocities (medical experimentation during Nazi Germany, the Tuskegee syphilis study, Milgram experiments and so on) and a whole series of less-famous national scandals (such as those documented in Pappworth [1967] and the Alder Hey organs scandal in the UK). Widely publicised abuses in research – combined with other factors, such as that research is a professionalised activity, which creates reputational concerns within institutions and organisations, and requires guidelines and regulations – created the impression that research is particularly risky and so requires especially close scrutiny and stringent regulation.

Non–Risk-Related Grounds for Research Exceptionalism

The second strategy for defending research exceptionalism is more promising. Perhaps research is not riskier than other sorts of activities, but, nonetheless, there are different reasons for which it should be more heavily regulated. This strategy is represented in the literature by Wilson and Hunter's (2010: 50–52) 'three better arguments for research exceptionalism': the benefits of research do not accrue to participants; research requires public trust; and research ethics decision making is complex. These 'better arguments' do not rely on the claim that research is particularly risky; rather, these are putative reasons for regulating research more strictly despite the fact that it is not riskier than other sorts of activities. To see how well they fare, take each in turn.

The first is that, 'benefits of research mostly accrue to others than those taking the risks of research' (Wilson and Hunter 2010: 50). Put in terms of risk, this sounds like another risk-related feature, so it would belong in the first strategy; but the point is not really about risk but about unjust distribution of burdens and benefits: research is distinctively unfair in burdening participants for the benefit of others. Wilson and Hunter are alert to the obvious objection that some research does benefit participants – for example, 'patients with chronic conditions, whose treatment next year may well benefit from knowledge gained in the randomised evaluations they participate in today' (van Staa et al. 2012) – and deal with it by saying that 'generally' research is neither intended to benefit nor actually benefits participants.

But there are stronger objections. John (2010) points out that everyone benefits *indirectly* from the 'social institution of research', a point which Hunter and Wilson (2010) take (and their rejoinder – 'we were primarily pointing towards the motivations and perceptions of the researcher' – is somewhat opaque). Furthermore, as Wendler (2017) put it, 'our everyday activities frequently expose some to risks for the benefit of others', so the asymmetry between burdens and benefits is hardly restricted to research, and we would not countenance subjecting these everyday activities to ethical scrutiny and strict regulation.

The second 'better argument for research exceptionalism' Wilson and Hunter canvass is that 'research is dependent on public trust', which is engendered by stringent regulation. This is akin to the last of four arguments for research exceptionalism discussed by Hansson (2011: 26) – the only one he finds 'plausible' – based on 'social standing and reputation of research'. That research relies on something like public trust is clearly true, but whether public trust is supported by closer ethical scrutiny is highly questionable. Since ethical oversight is by ethics committees, Wilson and Hunter seem to give the game away by admitting, 'most people outside of research have never heard of them'. But this could be a reason for better publicising research governance frameworks, including the work of ethics committees, as opposed to a fundamental objection to the argument. The stronger objection is that research is not exceptional in relying on trust. As John (2010: 68) points out, 'all social interactions [and] social practices' require trust, so reliance on public trust fails to distinguish research and, in turn, cannot justify closer scrutiny and stringent regulation.

Wilson and Hunter's third argument is that research exceptionalism is justified because research ethics is made complex by uncertainty inherent in research and the plurality of relevant values. The expertise and 'democratically set regulations' this complexity demands justify the special treatment of research, including ethics committee review as opposed to relying on individual researchers. One response to the argument is to question the premise; Wilkinson (2010: 64), for example, queries whether Wilson and Hunter 'overstate the uncertainty of research outcomes' and what they have in mind by appeals to 'democratic legitimacy and regulation'. But furthermore, research is hardly our only ethically complex practice. John (2010) presses this by drawing an analogy between research and religion, suggesting that Wilson and Hunter's argument tends in an illiberal direction by implying stricter state regulation of all practices that admit of ethical uncertainty and value pluralism. The analogy with religion is distracting – in their response, Hunter and Wilson (2010: W5–W6) prey on it, for example – as is the charge of illiberalism; but John's point that ethical complexity is not restricted to research, so cannot ground research exceptionalism, is surely right.

A Dialectical Pattern

A dialectical pattern has emerged from the discussion in this section. The question is whether research exceptionalism can be justified. Two strategies were suggested. In both, features of research are suggested which might justify research exceptionalism: risk related, in the first strategy, and risk independent – unjust distribution of burdens and benefits, public trust, and ethical complexity – in the second. There are problems specific to some of these suggestions; for example, participants do benefit from research, ethics committees do not engender public trust, and research is not that uncertain. But more to the point, there is a problem shared by all of them: none of the justifying features is unique to research, but is shared by lots of other activities and practices. This creates a general dilemma for defenders of research exceptionalism. Particularly close ethical scrutiny and stringent regulation of research are unjustified; or, if they are justified, then, to be consistent, so are close ethical scrutiny and stringent regulation of other activities which are alike in relevant respects, but which we neither do nor should regulate.

This failure to establish research exceptionalism is hardly surprising in light of the defence of the research–practice distinction in the previous chapter. In effect, both strategies discussed here are attempts to justify research exceptionalism by revealing the feature of research which makes it different from other activities in a way that justifies special oversight and stringent regulation. We already know this will not work. We know because the conceptual issue addressed in the previous chapter – whether research and practice can be distinguished – is driven precisely by the fact that there is no defining characteristic of research, no feature of all and only research. So we were bound to discover that any proposed feature of research is shared by other activities and, in turn, that it fails to justify research exceptionalism, on the one hand, and creates the dilemma just outlined on the other.

To refocus this discussion on public health, research exceptionalism in public health is even less plausible than research exceptionalism in general. Take, for example, the attempt to defend research exceptionalism on the grounds that participants do not benefit from research. This does not just fail in the public health context, it fails by definition. All public health information-gathering activities – whether research or some form of public health practice – aim by definition to benefit the public, not the individuals whose data are collected. So it is particularly stark that regulating research in public health more stringently than public health practice which gathers information, cannot be based on the fact that the former fails to benefit 'participants'. Likewise, recall the suggestion that research exceptionalism is justified on grounds of public trust. There is clearly no argument from public trust to regulating research and practice in public health differently, because trust is important across the board of these information-gathering activities: public health practice depends on public trust just as much as does any research activity (which is why it is the subject of chapter 7).

GOVERNANCE OF PUBLIC HEALTH INFORMATION

To summarise the discussion so far, the taxonomy of public health information presented in the last chapter made the research–practice distinction. This was defended by taking a broadly Wittgensteinian approach. So, there is no conceptual objection to the current system of regulating research more heavily than nonresearch activities (including public health practice). But this is a form of research exceptionalism, and the previous section established that research exceptionalism is unjustified in general, and is even less plausible in the public health context. This would seem to entail that there is no justification for treating research and nonresearch activities differently, so all information gathering should be under the purview of ethics and governance arrangements.

The last move is too quick, because it could be that, in the specific case of public health information, public health practice which generates data happens not to create any serious ethical issues. But the literature is awash with discussions of ethical problems that arise in the context of public health practices which gather and use data. A few from myriad examples will illustrate the point. The ethics of surveillance is the subject of major World Health Organization guidelines (WHO, 2017) and systematic reviews (Klingler et al. 2017). Ethics of data collection during emergencies and outbreaks are discussed in general (Mitra and Sethi 2016) and in the context of specific outbreaks, such as Ebola (Schopper et al. 2017). The sorts of service evaluation distinguished in the taxonomy – including audit (Wade 2005) and quality improvement (Baily et al. 2006) – have long been the subject of ethical discussion.

Likewise, the three sources of information for public health distinguished in the taxonomy clearly create ethical issues. Discussions of the ethics of health activity data have focused on electronic health records (Williams et al. 2015), aggregate health data (Matthews, Harel and Aseltine 2016) and distinctive forms of data, such as from neuroimaging (Brakewood and Poldrack 2013). Biobanks have been the subject of intense ethical scrutiny (Virani and Longstaff 2015). And there is burgeoning literature on the ethics of novel forms of health information garnered from Internet, social media, and online sharing platforms, both in general research (Golder et al. 2017) and in public health in particular (Conway 2014). The ethics of each 'cross-cutting themes' in the taxonomy – secondary analysis, data linkage and 'big data' – are also well represented in the literature: see, respectively, Tripathy 2013; Kelman, Bass and Holman (2002); Vayena et al. (2015).

Governance Inflation

Evidently, all categories in the taxonomy of public health information create ethical issues, so there is no objection to bringing all public health information under governance arrangements on the grounds that public health practice is not ethically relevant. But extending governance to public health practice implies more regulation of information-gathering activities; i.e. not only research, but public health practice too. And this is problematic in two respects.

First, extending governance to all public health information will massively increase the burden on regulatory mechanisms; in particular, ethics committees will be inundated with extra submissions by public health practitioners requiring review and approval. Second, extending governance arrangements to public health practice is hugely undesirable: public health is vitally important, and information is vital to public health, so we should be facilitating the acquisition and use of data, not extending the reach of governance to public health practice which currently escapes close scrutiny and extra regulation. In other words, if '[t]reating research differently is harmful to public health because it slows progress on solving important problems' (Rivera 2014: 55), how much slower will progress be when we stop treating research differently and scrutinise public health practice too? (For vivid accounts of the undesirability of extending governance to nonresearch activities, see Pronovost et al. 2006; Candib 2007.)

Basically, there is a dilemma. On the one hand, the current system of restricting oversight to all and only research is untenable in public health, because research exceptionalism is false and information-generating public health practice is ethically relevant. On the other hand, bringing all public health information under existing governance arrangements is impracticable and undesirable. But there are ways to navigate a way through this dilemma.

Overregulation of Research

The latter part of the dilemma assumes that current governance arrangements for research stay as they are, but in addition – and in order to be intellectually robust – public health information-gathering practices should be scrutinised and regulated as well. But a persistent theme in the literature is that research, including in the context of public health, is massively overscrutinised (Warlow 2005). This has motivated what Wilson and Hunter (2010: 45) call, 'a backlash against this apparent overregulation of research'. In turn, this suggests a straightforward strategy for bringing public health practice under the purview of governance in way that is practicable and desirable: scrutinise more practice but less research, and avoid overregulating either.

In pursuing this, the first thing to address is that the claim that research is overregulated is sometimes presented in the literature in ways that could be misconstrued. There are two versions of the overregulation claim: first, we scrutinise and regulate some research unnecessarily; second, we scrutinise and regulate research more than we do other activities. The first is clearly the important version of the claim, because the second version does not establish that research is overregulated; after all, the disparity in how much we regulate research compared to other activities might be justified (that we scrutinise planes more closely than other vehicles does not get us to overregulation of air travel, because the disparity is justified). But sometimes the overregulation claim is made in ways which might suggest this second version. For example, Wilson and Hunter (2010: 45) outline 'three responses we could make to this "overregulation" charge'. The third – 'research merits stringent regulation despite the fact that it is no riskier than many other activities' – was dealt with above, in the discussion of research exceptionalism, so is not relevant here. But the other two are:

> We could argue that we are too lax in the way we regulate various other activities and that we should regulate them more stringently to bring them into line with the way we regulate research. Second, we could argue that we are too stringent in the way we currently regulate research, and we should relax our research regulations to bring them into line with the way we regulate other activities.

Putting overregulation in terms of 'bringing activities into line' with one another suggests the second version of the claim, i.e. that the problem is the disparity in how much we regulate activities. In turn, this indicates that we solve the problem by achieving parity, either by regulating research less or nonresearch activities more. But to reiterate, it is the first version of the claim that is important: we regulate research unnecessarily, whether or not it is regulated 'in line with' other activities. A disparity in how much we regulate activities might alert us to the important sort of overregulation, but it is not the salient point.

The evidence that research is overregulated – in the relevant sense that there is unnecssary scrutiny – seems unassailable. There is a sizeable literature documenting overzealous oversight (Stewart et al. 2008; Snooks et al. 2012). Complaints of deleterious effects range from costly and lengthy overbureaucratic procedures, to consequences for specific research objectives, such as 'to reduce uncertainties about the effects of treatments already in use within "normal" or "usual" clinical practice' (Chalmers 2007). Related complaints are that research regulation is itself unevaluated and arbitrary (Davies, Wells and Czarkowski 2009; Bean 2010: 59). Mechanisms by which there is 'governance creep' towards overregulation are revealed; for example, Schwab (2010: 55) identifies 'three features of the federal regulations and their application' that explain the tendency in institutional review boards toward overreaching regulation.

That research is overregulated seems unassailable, but a point counting against the claim should be addressed. It is easy to demonstrate the failures of research governance, but not its success. As Bean (2010: 59) says of the current research regulatory schema: 'It is difficult to empirically verify counterfactuals such as the prevention of an adverse event [hence] the paucity of evidence to prove its usefulness' (see also Hunter and Wilson 2010: W4). In other words, we cannot quantify the success of research governance because successful systems stop bad things happening, and we cannot observe things that do not happen. Given this lack of evidence, we are unable to evaluate the regulatory schema, so we should suspend criticism.

But this is surely an unconvincing move. Bean does not take 'paucity of evidence' to disallow criticism of research regulation, and this seems right because the overregulation of research is egregious. For example, McCullough (2010) describes the tortuous process involved in getting approval for a study which 'did not pose even a risk of a paper cut'; and Rid (2014: 418) is one of many commentators to point out that 'in the U.S., 40–50% of new protocols submitted for REC review fall into the minimal risk category'. No amount of harping on the verifiability of counterfactuals can justify this sort of overregulation. Rather, there is a clear tendency to assume that all research *qua* research is equally very dangerous, so requires what McCullough decries as the 'one size fits all' approach to governance.

Given that research is overregulated, how should regulators and review bodies respond? There are lots of suggestions in the literature (Bean et al. 2010); but the more ambitious response is to devise a system of proportional review in which the sort and degree of scrutiny, and stringency of regulation, are commensurate with the ethical issues and level of risk of the study in question.

Proportional Review

Proportional review sounds uncomplicatedly promising. Proportionality is a well-established legal principle (Engle 2012), and the basic idea in the present context seems straightforward: screen projects for ethical risk, then triage studies by undertaking an appropriate review. As is often pointed out, the 'idea of proportionality is also already embedded in the ethics review process' (McGrail, Gutteridge and Meagher 2015: 748). In fact, though this is not so often recognised, proportional review is actually unavoidable because no reviewer – individual, committee or any other – spends exactly the same amount of time and energy on all projects, but inevitably and rightly apportions his or her attention, length of discussion and so on, according to the seriousness of ethical concerns raised by studies. There also seems to be a fairly straightforward hierarchy of reviews comprising three main strata – no review of ethically risk-free studies, some form of expedited review of low-risk projects and full ethics committee review of high-risk projects – and variants of each, such as Chair's Action to expedite some studies, subcommittees of main committees and so on.

But this is deceptively simple, and proportional review has been challenged in two main ways, one general and the other more specific. The general query is how ethical issues and risks raised by studies are to be identified and measured. Hunter (2007) presents four features of the regulatory landscape – questionable expertise, ethical complexity, theoretical pluralism and uncertainty – which combine to make it difficult to identify ethical issues. This problem would be ameliorated if the level of risk posed by studies mapped neatly onto something else, such as the distinction between types of enquiry or institutions; but the level of risk clearly varies independently of these, so there is no easy way to distinguish between studies in terms of risk (Hunter and Wilson 2010: W5). This creates a dilemma. On the one hand, risk screening could be done outside of a full ethics committee; this would achieve the aims of proportional review, but would threaten to misidentify ethical risk because only ethics committees are well placed to get this right. On the other hand, risk screening could be done by a full ethics committee; this is the surest way of correctly identifying ethical risk, but achieves none of the aims of proportional review.

The more specific way in which proportional review has been challenged centres on proposed criteria for triaging studies. A well-known suggestion dates back to the 2005 Warner Review of NHS RECs: 'The remit of NHS RECs should not include surveys or other nonresearch activity if they present *no material ethical issues* for human participants' (Department of Health 2005 [emphasis added]). Edwards and Omar (2008) query this by focusing on definitions of 'material'. Some candidates are clearly hopeless: circular definitions of 'material' as meaning 'serious', and question-begging definitions such as 'material issues' means 'legal issues', for example. Edwards and Omar pursue the more plausible interpretation of 'material ethical issues' in terms of risk, and appeal to the familiar US Code of Federal Regulations' (45 CFR 46.102) definition: 'Minimal risk means that the probability and magnitude of harm or discomfort anticipated in the research are not greater in and of themselves than those ordinarily encountered in daily life or during the performance of routine physical and psychological examinations or tests' (Code of Federal Regulations; see also Kopelman 2004). Nonetheless, suggest Edwards and Omar, proportional review is compromised by the remaining ambiguities and a lack of clarity around this 'minimal risk' account of 'material issues' (see also Yentis and Dawson 2006).

Ethical Risk Screening

It is argued here that such scepticism about proportional review is misplaced. For one thing, individual concerns of the kinds reported here can be met. The dilemma between 'efficiency and effectiveness' Hunter (2007: 244) describes surely misrepresents how difficult it is to identify ethically low-risk projects. In the context of a discussion of research exceptionalism, Wilson and Hunter (2010: 49) say: 'Much research – in particular a considerable amount of survey based research seems – barring the risk of a paper cut – almost entirely risk free'. This clearly indicates that it overstates the problem to suggest a full committee is required to identify ethical risks. Similarly, Edwards and Omar overstate the difficulty of giving substantive content to the notion of 'minimal risk'. For example, having introduced the concept, they immediately raise worries around objectivity and relativity (p. 569). But, for example, risks 'ordinarily encountered in daily life' are objective matters of fact – i.e. they exist independently of what people think or say about them – and that they are 'inevitably relative to context' does nothing to detract from their usefulness as a benchmark for purposes of proportional review (cf. Kim, Ubel and De Vries 2009).

But the best rejoinder is that such scepticism is belied by successful proportional review systems devised and refined specifically for public health information. An excellent example is the Public Health Ontario (PHO) Risk Screening Tool developed for the 'ethical appraisal of evidence-generating initiatives' in public health (Ondrusek et al. 2015). In passing, it is worth pointing out that Ondrusek et al. (2015) base the screening tool on the fact that, 'the boundary between [research and practice] is not clear, and attempts to develop criteria to reliably separate them have proven unsatisfactory'. As argued in the previous chapter, this is to mistake a vague boundary for no boundary, and to assume that the research-practice distinction requires a definition or criteria for these activities. But otherwise, the PHO Risk Screening Tool is precisely what we are looking for: 'systematic consideration of risks for all evidence-generating initiatives involving human participants, their biological material or their data, regardless of whether or not they are classified as "research", and to support a proportionate approach to ethics review based on risk rather than project type' (p. 3).

Crucially, the PHO Tool has been validated, tested and revised in an iterative fashion, and as the quote indicates, it is well-suited to the whole range of public health information categorised in the taxonomy presented in chapter 1 (see also Public Health Ontario 2012). Furthermore, it is not the only example of a convincing proportional review system in the public health field. For example, McGrail, Gutteridge and Meagher (2015) present a 'proportionate governance framework' for secondary data; and Cave and Nichols (2007) recommend extending regulatory oversight to clinical audit – including inaugurating Audit Ethics Committees – which sounds like governance inflation, except that Cave and Nichols provide details on how this would be achieved proportionately, including an appropriate triage system. Of course, the development of proportional review systems is ongoing, including comparative studies of 'risk-adaptive regulation', analysis of challenges and ethical concerns they raise, and iterations of 'risk-adaptive approaches' (Rid 2014). Nonetheless, progress made indicates that scepticism about proportional review is misplaced.

In sum, the position advocated here is that the current restriction of ethical oversight to research should be replaced by bringing all public health information under the purview of ethics and governance; and the impracticability and undesirability of extending governance from research to practice are to be avoided by developing proportional review systems which screen projects for ethical risks and review projects commensurately.

HOW SHOULD PUBLIC HEALTH INFORMATION GATHERING BE EVALUATED?

The discussion so far has centred on what to scrutinise and regulate, the answer being, all public health information–gathering activities, proportionately. As a coda to this chapter, how should these activities be evaluated? In one respect, the answer seems straightforward. We already have a rich understanding of research ethics and a well-developed research governance system, including a network of research ethics committees. These can simply be extended and adapted to incorporate public health evidence–generating initiatives. A case in point just encountered is Cave and Nichols's (2007) suggestion that if a clinical audit raises sufficient ethical concern to require scrutiny, it can be reviewed by an Audit Ethics Committee, equivalent to an existing research ethics committee. This can be broadened to cover other sorts of public health information gathering.

Distinctive Ethical Appraisal

But there is a less straightforward way of taking the question, not in terms of where public health evidence–generating initiatives are reviewed, but how they should be evaluated. A persistent theme in the literature is that public health, and the ethical issues it raises, are so distinctive as to require a different sort of ethical appraisal. This goes back to the start of public health ethics as a subdiscipline. In a seminal piece, for example, Callahan and Jennings (2002: 169) suggest: 'Public health raises a number of moral problems that extend beyond the earlier boundaries of bioethics and require their own form of ethical analysis'. Callahan and Jennings were writing about public health in general, but one of the examples they give (p. 171) is 'epidemiology and other public health research':

> Research with human subjects has been a central ethical problem for biomedicine for at least 100 years, but particularly since World War II. Yet, is the biomedical model – focused on individual informed consent and tightly regulated research with those at risk of exploitation – an appropriate model for public health, one that may either pose no medical or other risks to individuals or make consent impractical to gain in research encompassing large communities?

This is part of a larger theme, and arises in the context of public health practice as well as research studies. Prior to Callahan and Jennings' piece, Gostin (1991:191) 'provides a halting first step in organizing a set of ethical guidelines for the conduct of population based research, surveillance and practice' (see also Burris, Buehler and Lazzarini 2003). Subsequently, Buchanan and Miller (2006) took a 'public health perspective on research ethics'; and Verweij and Dawson (2009), in a piece that deserved more attention, tried to motivate a 'public health research ethics agenda' by attempting 'to clarify, analyse and discuss the most pressing moral problems in public health research ethics, rather than focus on trying to perfect a set of regulation' (p. 3; although overly focused on a *research* agenda, Verweij and Dawson (2009) – and other papers in that volume – discuss other evidence-generating practices, such as surveillance, data linkage and collection during public health emergencies).

What motivates this theme is straightforward and frequently alluded to in the relevant literature. Research ethics, regulation and governance developed during the postwar period in response to studies which were egregiously abusive of individual participants; i.e. research's 'checkered past', mentioned in the previous discussion of research exceptionalism, including a familiar litany of infamy: Nazi atrocities, Tuskegee and so on. So, standard research ethics, regulation and governance are geared to clinical trials and human experiments – because these created the scandals – and focus on protecting the rights and interests of individual participants, because these were scandalously ignored. Hence the emphasis on voluntary informed consent (to respect participants' autonomy), confidentiality (to protect their information), equipoise (to ensure no one is denied the best known treatment), just distributions of burdens and benefits (to avoid exploitation) and such like. Constraints on research to protect participants were reiterated and refined in policy documents including, for example, supranational – such as the Helsinki Declaration (1964) and Belmont Report (1979) – and national legislation (for example, the UK Research Governance Framework, which has been reconstructed since 2001) and regulation of specific aspects of research such as the UK's Human Tissue Act (2004) and Mental Capacity Act (2005).

Given this background, it is clear that standard research ethics, regulation and governance are ill-suited to public health evidence–generating initiatives. As the taxonomy of public health information in the previous chapter shows, most public health information is gathered not by clinical trials or human experiments, but by activities such as surveillance, service evaluations and secondary data analysis, which do not involve recruiting individual participants. In fact, even some standard forms of public health research, which share methodologies with clinical trials, do not recruit individual participants. For example, in cluster randomised trials, collectives (such as health care units, including primary care facilities or general practitioner practices) as opposed to individual participants are randomised to each arm of the trial (Weijer et al. 2011). So, given how standard research ethics, regulation and governance developed, they are bound to provide an imperfect template for the evaluation of public health information–gathering activities; hence the calls for a novel 'form of ethical analysis' – or a new perspective or agenda – for public health data collection.

Identifying verses Weighing Considerations

There is clearly a lot to be said for this line of thought, but the crucial question is, how and to what extent should the evaluation of public health information–gathering activities diverge from standard research ethics, regulation and governance? This can be framed in terms of how radically to interpret the suggestion that public health information requires a different sort of ethical analysis. To answer this requires an account of what evaluation of information-gathering activities comprises.

Evaluation consists of identifying and weighing relevant considerations in order to arrive at a balanced judgement. To illustrate, a standard research ethics committee's evaluation of a nonpublic health research project would include identifying considerations relevant to that project, weighing them relative to one another, then deciding whether the study can be approved. For example, in reviewing a project, a research ethics committee might identify deception of and benefits to participants as key considerations, weigh these against one another, and judge that the minor deception is outweighed by the significant benefits, so approve the study.

The first thing to note is that suggestions such as, 'moral problems in public health require their own form of ethical analysis', or that evaluation of public health evidence–generating initiatives requires a new perspective or agenda, cannot be as radical as to suggest a form of evaluation other than the process of identifying and weighing considerations just sketched. There really is no viable alternative to this process. So, whatever such suggestions amount to will involve a shift in emphasis as opposed to dismantling the familiar fundamental process of evaluation.

The important point is that this process of evaluation has two components: identifying and weighing considerations. So, calls for a novel form of ethical analysis of public health information–gathering activities are ambiguous between these two components of evaluation. On one reading, these suggestions would be met when considerations distinctive of public health, which might otherwise go missing, are identified. On the other reading, public health gets 'its own form of ethical analysis' not just by identifying considerations which are distinctive of public health, but by weighing those considerations particularly heavily; in particular, heavily enough to outweigh competing considerations. The position taken here is that the former of these readings is fine, but the latter is highly questionable.

To take each in turn, public health information is a domain of information within which distinctive considerations arise. Of course, standard considerations which are familiar from other sorts of information gathering arise too – the acceptability of recruitment methods (Sifunda et al. 2014), whether potential harms to participants are outweighed by the benefits of the research (Bambery et al. 2016), how to deal with incidental findings (Merritt 2016), and so on – but the important point for present purposes is that evidence-generating initiatives in public health create additional distinctive considerations. Mainly, this is due to the distinctive goals of public health, but also in part due to its idiosyncratic information-gathering activities, such as community-based participatory research (Shore 2006).

Relevant considerations are distinctive of public health information in two respects. First, familiar considerations are given a 'public health twist'. For example, trading-off harms and benefits is very familiar, but distinctive sorts of harms and benefits arise in the context of public health information: 'In public health . . . researchers focus on the well-being of communities' (Mikesell, Bromley and Khodyakov 2013). Second, considerations unique to public health evidence gathering arise, including social justice concerns, such as reducing health inequalities, and communal values, for example, protecting communities and promoting solidarity.

Evaluating public health information–gathering activities should be informed by these distinctive considerations. Referring back to the theme in the literature traced above, distinctive considerations come into focus by taking Buchanan and Miller's (2006) 'public health perspective on research ethics', or distinctive considerations are new items on Verweij and Dawson's (2009) 'public health research ethics agenda'. So to this extent, evidence-generating initiatives in public health should get what Callahan and Jennings (2002) call their 'own form of ethical analysis'. Conversely, to impose standard ways of evaluating evidence-generating initiatives threatens to ignore these distinctive public health considerations and thereby distort the evaluation.

But some commentators advocate not only identifying distinctively public health considerations, but also the more radical suggestion that such considerations are weighed more heavily. For example, Östlin et al. (2011) proposed a 'paradigm shift in health research' from traditional clinical research objectives to an equity-focused agenda. This clearly goes beyond erstwhile more measured commitment to achieving public health goals – such as, 'at times, minimizing preexisting social injustices' (Kass 2001) – in suggesting that equity is an overriding consideration. Likewise, McMillan (2011), in 'considering the appropriate normative framework for public health research' suggests nonexploitation as the 'new principle for population-based research ethics' (p. 174). This is implausible (exploitation is hardly 'new') but, more to the point, it is another example of going beyond merely identifying distinctively public health considerations, to weighing them more heavily. Suppose, for example, a public health evidence–generating initiative would significantly reduce health inequalities or exploit a vulnerable population; not only would these be identified as considerations to be weighed, they would also weigh heavily when evaluating the project, and might well outweigh competing considerations. This extra step, from merely identifying to weighing more heavily public health considerations, is deeply problematic.

The basic problem is that it begs the evaluative question as to whether an information-gathering activity is justified, by assuming that it is, just because it conduces to the goals of that sort of activity. To see this, note that it begs the evaluative question in precisely the opposite way in which standard research ethics and governance do: whereas standard research ethics and governance would distort evaluation by assuming the most important thing is to protect the rights and interests of individual participants – this being the *raison d'être* of standard research ethics, regulation and governance, as already outlined – this novel 'form of ethical analysis' for public health distorts evaluation by assuming the most important thing is reducing health inequalities or promoting social solidarity or whatever. More generally, it is clearly dubious to allow partisan evaluation, i.e. evaluation of activities that assumes the activities are justified just if they conduce to the goals of the activity in question. Evaluation should be more objective, and less biased in favour of preferred goals, than this. In sum, evaluation of public health evidence–generating initiatives should diverge from the standard only to the extent of identifying distinctive considerations, but not to the extent of weighing those considerations differently in favour of public health goals.

Chapter 3

Privacy

It was argued in the previous chapter that all public health information–gathering activities categorised in the taxonomy in chapter 1 are under the purview of ethics and governance. At this point, the discussion could be continued in a number of directions. One option is to go through each sort of activity – research, surveillance, service evaluation, etc. – discussing the ethical issues it raises and recommending regulatory and governance responses. But this piecemeal approach would be unsatisfying, because there are fundamental themes shared by all public health evidence–generating initiatives; better, then, to identify and address those themes, judiciously applying findings to individual information-gathering activities.

Privacy is the value fundamental to the ethics and governance of public health information–gathering activities. This is masked by frequent references in relevant literature to several cognate concepts. In particular, apart from privacy, it is typical for concerns about public health information to be put in terms of consent, confidentiality and trust (see Lee, Heilig and White 2012; Williams et al. 2015; Platt and Kardia 2015, respectively). But although these concepts are cognate, privacy is fundamental. The point of consent is to protect privacy by controlling access to one's personal information; confidentiality ensures privacy by restricting further disclosures of private information; and we need to trust institutions to manage our information in ways that respect our privacy. Conversely, without privacy concerns, the requirements of consent, confidentiality and trust would fall away. This is not to say that such requirements are unimportant – nor to decry sustained analyses of them – but nonetheless, of these cognate concepts, privacy is fundamental.

Privacy is also fundamental to the overall aim of this book, as set out in the Introduction. To recall, the problematic is the privacy-utility dilemma as it plays out in the informational domain of public health. The aim is to defend public health information from the discernible tendency to prioritise privacy protection over social utility. In this chapter, a dualistic account of privacy is presented and defended. This will allow us to precisely identify the specific sort of privacy concerns which arise in public health, including revealing how privacy concerns about public health data are exaggerated. To begin the argument, how should privacy be analysed?

ANALYSING PRIVACY

There is a huge literature on privacy, very little by way of agreement, and it would be overambitious to attempt to resolve this here (DeCew 2018). Nonetheless, there is space for the more modest project of sketching an account of privacy as it applies specifically to public health information. First, how should the concept of privacy be approached? There is a persistent tendency in the literature to analyse privacy by focusing on legal protection of privacy rights, based on an early treatise by legal scholars (Warren and Brandeis [1890] is a *locus classicus*). This is not the best approach, for numerous reasons.

The basic problem is that privacy rights are legal entities established and protected in specific privacy laws within a given legislative system; an example is privacy rights protected by UK laws governing press intrusion, which are under seemingly constant review. So, starting with legal privacy rights has various ramifications. A fairly straightforward implication is the tendency to confuse the descriptive and the normative, i.e. 'descriptive accounts of privacy, describing what is in fact protected as private, from normative accounts of privacy defending its value and the extent to which it should be protected' (DeCew 2018). The two are obviously connected – laws are intended to protect what is valuable – but in the present context of a discussion of ethics and governance of public health information, the normative account, not the descriptive account, is relevant.

There is a more serious but subtler ramification of starting an account of privacy with privacy rights enshrined in privacy laws. Rights theory is concerned with identifying, defining and clarifying the interrelations between rights. So talk of a legally protected right to privacy invites an enquiry into whether this putative right exists and, if so, what it amounts to, and how it relates to other rights. It would be unsurprising if such an enquiry took a sceptical turn. A famous example is Thomson (1975), who starts with: 'Perhaps the most striking thing about the right to privacy is that nobody seems to have any very clear idea what it is' (p. 295). Thomson's thesis is that,

> the right to privacy is 'derivative' in this sense: it is possible to explain in the case of each right in the [right to privacy] cluster how come we have it without ever once mentioning the right to privacy. Indeed, the wrongness of every violation of the right to privacy can be explained without ever once mentioning it (p. 313).

Although this sounds straightforwardly sceptical about the right to privacy, there is a complication. DeCew (2018) calls Thomson's 'the most famous reductionist view of privacy'. Reductionism is the process of analysing a complex phenomenon in terms of its simpler or more fundamental constituents. In this case, the complex phenomenon is the right to privacy; Thomson analyses this in terms of a cluster of other rights, so hers is a reductionist analysis. The complication is about what happens to the right to privacy – the explanandum – at the end of the analysis.

Generally, reductionism is ambiguous between realist and antirealist accounts of the explanandum (i.e. the complex phenomenon under analysis). In other words, the analysed phenomenon may or may not survive the reductive analysis and continue to exist (Kemeny and Oppenheim 1956; van Riel and Van Gulick 2018). This general ambiguity seems to arise in the present case: a realist reductionist analysis of the right to privacy would explain that right in terms of other rights, but leave it intact; whereas an antirealist reductionist analysis would eliminate the right to privacy by replacing it with Thomson's 'cluster' of other rights. And the former option – the realist version which preserves the right to privacy – sounds less sceptical than the latter, which amounts to eliminativism about the right to privacy.

But the prospect of a realist reductionist analysis does not really salvage the strategy of starting an account of privacy with a putative right to privacy as protected in law. Although she was typically nuanced, Thomson's view is always taken to be that 'there is no right to privacy' (DeCew 2018) and that she 'denies that there is such a thing as *the* right to privacy' (Scanlon 1975: 315). And whether or not this is the correct reading of Thomson, eliminativism about the right to privacy is explicit elsewhere: 'This paper is an inquiry into the formation and possible disintegration of a legal concept, right of privacy, inviting comparison with the life history of a scientific concept like "ether" or "atom"' (Freund 1971: 182). Furthermore, philosophical analyses of privacy which start with a legal right to privacy end up sceptical: 'Few philosophers would argue that privacy is a "natural" right or that the intrinsic nature of privacy establishes it as a legal right' (Negley 1966: 319). Evidently, starting with a putative right to privacy enshrined in law leads to scepticism and eliminativism.

Worse still, reductionism and scepticism about privacy *qua* legal right, slides over into scepticism about privacy as a concept, or as a distinctive set of concerns and interests; for example, 'any *interest* protected as private can be equally well explained and protected by other interests or rights . . . what are called *privacy concerns* [are] analyzable or reducible to claims of other sorts' (DeCew 2018 [emphases added]). Likewise, Bloustein (1964: 962) imputes William Posser with the view that, 'privacy is not an independent value at all but rather a composite of the interests in reputation, emotional tranquility and intangible property'. The endpoint of this line of thought is nicely summarized by Moore (2007: 814):

> Reductivists argue that privacy is derived from other rights such as life, liberty, and property rights; there is no overarching concept of privacy but, rather, several distinct core notions that have been lumped together. Viewing privacy in this fashion might mean jettisoning the idea altogether and focusing on more fundamental concepts.

So, the really serious ramification of starting an account of privacy with privacy rights enshrined in privacy laws is that it threatens to do away not only with legal privacy rights but with privacy altogether.

A DUALIST ACCOUNT OF PRIVACY

Eliminating privacy not only sounds absurd, it is belied by a plausible substantive account of privacy. Given the morass of relevant literature, it would be unfeasible and, frankly, unwelcome to attempt anything like a full theory of privacy. But the aim here is the much more modest one of providing an account of privacy as it applies to public health information–gathering activities.

In light of the preceding discussion, this account starts not with the putative legal right to privacy. Rather, we should start with the concept of privacy and, in particular, the interests and concerns which come under the concept. The claim here is that, whatever else is true of privacy, two sorts of concerns or interests are captured by the concept. The first is best introduced metaphorically. Privacy is a matter of building personal space into the architecture of our lives. This is often put in terms of a private zone or sphere or territory which is required for us to enjoy valuable experiences, such as solitude and intimacy. The second sort of privacy concern is to protect personal information. Each of us has a privacy interest in maintaining control over who has access to facts about oneself; alongside this is the concern to control how personal information, once accessed, is used by others. So, the way to understand privacy is as referring to two sorts of interests, called here personal and informational, respectively.

An illustration will help to elucidate and establish the distinction. Imagine a couple having a restaurant meal. It is a private affair. The suggestion here is that 'private affair' covers two sorts of privacy interests. Literally and metaphorically, the couple need personal space. If the restaurant happens to be overcrowded and a stranger pulls up a chair at their table, their privacy interest in protecting their personal space is frustrated, and the occasion is ruined. Intimate conversation is no longer possible, for example. The couple might protect this privacy interest by refusing the stranger a place at their table. Second, information of various sorts will be generated by the occasion. This will range from the seemingly anodyne – who ordered what, for example – to the views and opinions, memories, hopes, desires and plans of the sort intended to be shared only between the couple. They might protect this privacy interest by lowering their voices during the meal so as not to disclose intimacies or personal information.

To reiterate, this is not an attempt at a complete theory of privacy. Nonetheless, the claim that there are two sorts of privacy interests is substantive. Generally, it amounts to saying that a complete theory of privacy must accommodate this distinction; conversely, a putative complete theory is vulnerable to a *reductio ad absurdum* objection if it repudiates the distinction. In particular, this distinction between two sorts of privacy interests does a lot of work later in the argument of this chapter, so it has to be defended.

THE PRIVACY LITERATURE

One way to defend and further elucidate the claim that privacy refers to two sorts of interests is to map it onto the sizeable body of privacy-related literature. The two privacy concerns distinguished here – personal and informational – figure prominently and repeatedly in analyses of privacy, both as theoretical claims and in innumerable illustrations (DeCew 2018). Classic legal scholarship on privacy made the distinction: for example, Westin (1967) says privacy allows for 'respite from the emotional stimulation of daily life' and to be 'always "on" would destroy the human organism', and that privacy 'is the claim of individuals, groups, or institutions to determine for themselves when, how, and to what extent information about them is communicated to others'. In his response to Thomson's scepticism, Rachels (1975: 326) distinguishes 'our ability to control who has access to us and to information about us'; the former is a personal privacy concern, the latter an informational privacy concern. And Calo's (2011: 1153) analysis of privacy harms is essentially dualistic: 'privacy harms fall into two distinct but meaningfully related categories . . . the subjective perception of unwanted observation or the unanticipated or coerced use of a person's information against them' (though Calo thinks of personal privacy as related to a 'subjective category of privacy harm', i.e. 'internal to the mind of the victim', whereas informational privacy is 'objective' in the sense of 'external' (p. 1133), which is not part of the dualistic account presented here).

Obfuscation

Despite frequent allusions to each sort of privacy interest, the distinction between them is often obscured in privacy literature, in various ways. One problem is the well-established practice of introducing and defending analyses of privacy by reference to more or less realistic scenarios and thought experiments in which privacy is violated. These tend to obscure the distinction between personal and informational privacy, because typical privacy violations frustrate both sorts of privacy interests at the same time. Incursions into one's personal space directly result in disclosure of personal information and, conversely, disclosure of personal information usually requires incursion into one's personal space. Take, for example, the standard case of bugging a couple's bedroom. This is ambiguous between a violation of one's privacy interest in maintaining a personal space (someone must have planted the bug) and in protecting personal information (listeners find out personal things). Likewise, in the earlier illustration, the stranger who sits in on the meal invades the couple's personal space and finds out intimate details about them. Since in such cases both sorts of privacy interests are frustrated, they are not conducive to making and maintaining a clear distinction between personal and informational privacy (Rachels 1975: 325).

Another possible source of obfuscation is the tendency for some writers to focus exclusively on one or other of the two sorts of privacy concerns. For example, in a long series of contributions, Moore (2003, 2007) offers a sustained analysis of informational privacy. By contrast, in another response to Thomson's sceptical account, Scanlon (1975) concentrates on the other sort of privacy concern, personal privacy, which he refers to as a 'zone' or 'territory' of privacy. Focusing a discussion on one of two privacy concerns threatens to collapse dualism into monism, i.e. reduce privacy concerns from two to one. This occurs when analyses are inattentive to the privacy concern not under scrutiny; for example, it seems odd of Moore (2007: 829–30) to characterise a 'garden-variety peeping Tom case' as being essentially about 'acquisition of information'. And sometimes a collapse into monism seems explicit. For example, Clarke (2006) relies on a working definition of privacy as, 'the interest that individuals have in sustaining a "personal space", free from interference by other people and organisations', which seems clearly to reduce privacy to personal privacy concerns at the expense of informational privacy.

Proliferation of Privacy Interests

Neither of these two forms of obfuscation are particularly serious: thought experiments can be read with the distinction between personal and informational privacy interests in mind, and exclusive focus on one privacy concern is fine, provided the other is acknowledged. But there is a more serious way the distinction between personal and informational privacy interests is obscured. This is by unnecessary proliferation, which happens in two main ways.

First, taxonomies of privacy duplicate privacy interests. A couple of specific examples illustrate the general phenomenon. Gostin (1991: 196) claims that the 'concept of privacy is as complicated as human affect itself' (see below for further illustrations of this exaggerated view of privacy's complexity) and suggests 'a right to privacy on three levels':

> The right to have space in the physical, personal or social sense (e.g. the absence of intrusive surveillance or questioning); a right to control the disclosure of information about their health, behavior or life circumstances (e.g. sexual or drug use history); and the right to maintain intimacy and confidences in their personal, family or social relationships (e.g. their interactions with sexual partners, spouses and professional counselors).

Leaving aside the rights talk – as previously recommended here – the first two of these concerns are about personal space and information, respectively; but the third is superfluous because it has been covered by the first two; so privacy interests have proliferated.

Duplication is even more obvious in taxonomies of privacy more complex than Gostin's. Finn et al. (2013) suggest 'seven types of privacy'; but admitting that these 'may have some overlaps' (p. 7), and that one 'might question what the difference is between privacy of location and space and privacy of behaviour' (p. 9), is tantamount to recognising duplications of interests in their list. Similarly, Rueben et al. (2017) present a four-fold taxonomy including sixteen subdivisions. Again, duplication is clear: they define privacy 'in terms of one's personal space or territory' *and* 'being physically removed from other people', for example; and what they call physical and social space should be conflated.

Category Errors

The other way in which privacy concerns are allowed to proliferate beyond personal and informational interests involves two sorts of category errors. Again, some specific illustrations will make the general point. The first sort of category error is to confuse privacy itself with privacy-related features:

> Many commentators have spoken of privacy as a unitary *concept* with a uniform value, which is unvarying across different situations. In contrast, I have argued that privacy *violations* involve a variety of types of harmful or problematic activities (Solove 2006: 480–481; [emphases added]).

Solove goes on to list six of the myriad ways in which privacy can be violated in order to bolster the claim that the 'concept of "privacy" is far too vague' (p. 482). But there is a clear slide here from the concept of privacy to violations of privacy. This is like attempting a definition of the concept of murder by listing all the ways people can kill each other. And just as 'murder' is a perfectly straightforward concept (unjustified killing of another human being) with lots of ways of performing murder, the fact that there are lots of ways of violating privacy does not make the concept 'far too vague'. This is not just a problem involving violations. The general tendency is to confuse definitions of privacy – which should focus on privacy concerns (of which there are two) – with related but nongermane features, such as the various reasons for which privacy is valued, ways in which it can be protected, effects of intrusions and so; since each of these is very varied, the impression is created that privacy itself is very complex, which is not the case.

The second sort of category error is to define privacy by mixing up privacy interests with concerns of other sorts, such as autonomy. For example, Kupfer (1987) proposed that 'privacy is a necessary condition for something of basic value – the development of an autonomous self'. Whether or not Kupfer gets the relation between privacy and autonomy right, his comment indicates that they are separate concerns, because something can only be a necessary condition of something else. But others have been tempted to confuse privacy and autonomy. For example, Rössler (2005) argues that there are three 'dimensions of privacy . . . decisional, informational and local'. Informational privacy is fine – and the 'local' dimension of privacy equates to personal privacy interests – but a 'decisional' dimension is questionable. Decisional privacy is usually defined in terms of the autonomy or freedom to make and act upon choices; this is obviously important, and privacy might be necessary for this, but autonomy and freedom are distinct from privacy. Including members of one category of value – autonomy or freedom, in this illustration – in the category of privacy is erroneous and overcomplicates the analysis of privacy (see also Resnik 2018: 149; Kahn 2003: 384–386; Calo 2011: 1136).

Exaggerated Complexity

Proliferating privacy concerns beyond personal and informational encourages the view that privacy is a massively complex phenomenon and a seemingly impossible concept to analyse. The privacy literature is awash with comments such as: 'The notion of privacy remains out of the grasp of every academic chasing it' (Gutwirth 2002: 31), and 'scholars have a famously difficult time pinning down the meaning of such a widely used term [and] most introduce their work by citing this difficulty' (Kasper 2005: 72). Such comments are as frequent as they are unchallenged and find a particularly strident expression in Solove's highly influential work; for example, his book *Understanding Privacy* starts with a chapter called 'Privacy: A Concept in Disarray':

> Nobody can articulate what it means. Currently, privacy is a sweeping concept, encompassing (among other things) freedom of thought, control over one's body, solitude in one's home, control over personal information, freedom from surveillance, protection of one's reputation, and protection from searches and interrogations. Philosophers, legal theorists, and jurists have frequently lamented the great difficulty in reaching a satisfying conception of privacy (Solove 2008: 1; see also Solove 2006).

This view that privacy means too many things to be pinned down is an exaggeration that can be traced to obfuscation and proliferation of the sorts already outlined. In fact, privacy is a straightforward concept which refers to two concerns of ours, namely, to enjoy personal space and protect personal information.

Privacy as a Family Resemblance Concept

This exaggerated view that privacy is a complex and elusive concept has predictably invited the suggestion that 'privacy is best understood as a family resemblance concept' (Solove 2006: 486; see also Solove 2002). Since this echoes the suggestion made in chapter 1 that research and practice are family resemblance concepts, it might be expected to be received sympathetically here. But there is a long-standing dispute over the question 'How far does the idea of family resemblance extend – to how many concepts does it apply?' (McGinn 2011: 14), to which there is a wide range of answers, broadly, from none to some to all (see, respectively, McGinn 2011; Sluga 2006; Ma and van Brakel 2016). Of these, that there are no family resemblance concepts is obviously not recommended here, given the claim in chapter 1 that research and practice are family resemblance concepts. Conversely, that all general concepts are family resemblance concepts seems intuitively implausible; given the diversity of our concepts, it would be surprising if any one treatment was appropriate to them all. Intuitively, the middle ground seems most plausible, i.e. different concepts work in different ways, some being fairly straightforward and easily defined by necessary and sufficient conditions, whilst other are so complex and elusive as to be family resemblance concepts. Certainly, that is what motivates specific claims, such as that art or religion, power, species and so on are family resemblance concepts; after all, such claims would be redundant if all concepts are family resemblance concepts.

Given this, the position taken here is that research is, and privacy is not, a family resemblance concept. To fully defend this view is not possible, but it requires some substantiating in order to dispel the worry that it is an arbitrary or ad hoc distinction. The main point to note is that the puzzle about research versus practice invites the 'family resemblance' move in a way that analyses of 'privacy' do not. To recall, we make and employ the research–practice distinction; this gets challenged precisely because there is nothing true of all and only research, i.e. no set of necessary and sufficient conditions for an activity being research. This is exactly what starts the Wittgensteinian line of thought about 'games' which ends with family resemblance concepts. But having clarified that privacy simply refers to two familiar and easily distinguished concerns – personal and informational – there is no equivalent motivation for thinking of it as a family resemblance concept. In fact, as outlined above, and illustrated by Solove's position, it is only by exaggerating the difficulty of defining privacy that one is misled into thinking that privacy is so complex and elusive that it must be a family resemblance concept. (Calo 2011: 1139–42 also responds to Solove's appeal to Wittgenstein; but Calo misinterprets Solove as using family resemblance to defend 'a list or taxonomy of privacy harms', whereas the point of the appeal is to avoid this sort of taxonomical approach.)

The Privacy Paradox

There is a different sort of objection to the dualist account of privacy proposed here discernible in the privacy literature. Our attitude to privacy is changing due to technological advances, notably, ubiquitous use of the Internet and social media. Changing privacy attitudes are the subject of a burgeoning interdisciplinary literature which is revealing important themes. For example, the 'privacy paradox' refers to the dissonance between what people say about privacy and their actual behaviours – notably, the anxiety people voice about privacy is belied by their willingness to share personal information – and interesting demographic disparities in privacy attitudes are emerging, such as intergenerational and between genders (Dowd 2010; López, Marín and Calderón, 2015; Solove 2008: 5). This might seem to be the basis of a challenge to the dualistic account of privacy presented here: the rapidity and extent of changes in privacy attitudes is not accommodated by the seemingly simplistic dualist account.

But this is a mistake. There is no doubt that there are massive changes taking place relating to privacy. But, once again, we need to distinguish the concept or definition of privacy from other privacy-related features. Changes in privacy attitudes relate to the latter, and do not impact on the former. To illustrate: 'As technological advancements are made, new means of both violating and protecting privacy may emerge and this is why technological developments are often met with concerns and questions relating to privacy' (Dowd 2010: 78). As this clearly indicates, the changes in privacy attitudes Dowd reveals are to do with 'new means of violating and protecting privacy', as opposed to privacy itself. And no doubt these are changing both rapidly and extensively. In turn, the innumerable new ways in which privacy can be invaded due to technological advances, and commensurably, many new forms of privacy protection, have an attitudinal effect. But none of that disturbs the dualistic analysis of the concept of privacy presented here. Recall a previous analogy, murder. As technology develops there are myriad new ways in which people can kill each other; this changes murder-related features, such as our means of protection, legislation and so on; in turn, this influences murder-related attitudes (we feel less secure, for example). Nonetheless, the concept of murder remains the same throughout: murder is still the unjustified killing of another human being.

What muddies these waters is that studies of privacy attitudes are persistently ambiguous between revealing changes in privacy-related features and privacy itself. For example, as mentioned, Dowd (2010) starts clearly enough, focusing on 'violating and protecting privacy'; but in a later section on 'conceptualising privacy', he goes on to say that his research 'does not rely on any predetermined, overarching conception of privacy but instead takes an approach which builds on the work of Solove' (p. 82). Inevitably, Dowd then traces Solove's line of thought from the exaggeratedly complex and elusive concept of privacy ('historically and culturally contingent . . . 'elastic' concept . . . vast number of ways in which it has been conceptualized' and so on) to advocating that privacy is a family resemblance concept. This line of thought – which is by no means restricted to Dowd (see also López, Marín and Calderón, 2015: 249) – was previously critiqued, so enquiries into changing privacy attitudes would do better to clearly focus on privacy-related matters – such as new ways of protecting and violating privacy – and resist the segue from changes in these to claiming that privacy itself is changing.

PRIVACY, FLOURISHING AND CONSEQUENCES

A dualistic account of privacy has been presented, centring on the distinction between a personal privacy interest in protecting one's private space and an informational privacy concern to control access to information about oneself.

This account has been defended and elucidated by reference to the privacy literature. To reiterate, this is not intended as a full defence; amongst other things, that would require more about how familiar privacy concerns – for example, about access to one's body or having private thoughts and opinions – can be subsumed under the two privacy interests, personal and informational, distinguished here. Nonetheless, this analysis is enough to continue the argument about public health information. To develop this, what is the relative importance of these two sorts of privacy concerns, for personal space and informational control? In this section it is argued that whilst both sorts of privacy interests are important, they are important for different reasons, such that our privacy interest in maintaining personal space is typically more important than informational privacy.

Flourishing versus Consequences

The way our personal privacy interest in maintaining a private space was introduced clearly indicates that it is grounded in a deep human need to enjoy certain experiences, such as solitude and intimacy. Privacy of this sort is a feature of flourishing and is constitutive of well-being or the good life for a human being. Life without a space to retreat to alone is a life without solitude, and a life without a zone or sphere exclusive to one's loved ones is a life without intimacy; and either is intolerable. All this might sound overblown. In fact, there is very strong empirical evidence from anthropological and zoological studies that personal privacy is as deeply important as is claimed here.

Starting with anthropology, it has long been established that personal privacy is a universal phenomenon, albeit one that is manifested differently between cultures. Altman (1977), for example, conceptualising privacy as 'selective control of access to the self', shows that 'privacy is a universal process that involves culturally unique regulatory mechanisms'. This is bolstered by anthropological explanations as to why privacy matters. For example, in a classic piece, Schwartz (1968) explained the universality of privacy by making reference to social benefits, such as being group preserving whilst maintaining status divisions. Well-known zoological studies also support the view that personal privacy is deeply important, including evidence that all animals seek seclusion, and that the lack of private space is a threat to survival (Westin 1967; Moore 2007).

By contrast, our privacy interest in controlling personal information is important not because of anything as grandiose as flourishing, well-being or the good life for a human being. There are no calls to see this as a fundamental part of human nature grounded in anthropological or zoological evidence. To take a banal example, animal studies will never reveal the depth of our interest in informational privacy because nonhuman animals such as rats are not creatures that produce, gather or use information. What grounds informational privacy concerns are potential adverse consequences of disclosures. The acquisition and use of facts about us by others incur risks of harm, ranging from embarrassment or distress, to being put at risk of disapprobation, uncomfortable exposure, financial ruin or prosecution. Hence there is a need to manage risk by controlling personal information, in terms of both who acquires it and how others use it. In sum, our privacy concern to protect personal space is a matter of flourishing, whereas our privacy concern to control personal information is consequentialist.

Objections

One possible objection to this is that both sorts of privacy interests are consequentialist; after all, what makes incursions into one's personal space bad are adverse effects, notably, loss of solitude or a reduced capacity for intimacy. What is right about this objection is that failure to meet either privacy interest – personal or informational – is intolerable; an entirely public life lacking privacy in the sense of personal space would be intolerable, and it would be intolerable for everyone to know everything about oneself, and to be able to deploy that knowledge in any way at all. But the objection obscures an important distinction by trading on the fact that any value or good can be described in consequentialist terms. In other words, any value or good can be said to be important because its absence or loss would be a bad consequence (in this case, personal space is important because to lose it would have deleterious effects on our well-being). We should resist this reductionism and maintain the insight that personal and informational privacy are important on different grounds, or for different reasons, namely, flourishing and consequences, respectively.

Another possible objection is that informational privacy interests are not solely, and perhaps not even mainly, consequentialist in nature. This is based on the familiar fact that people do not like certain sorts of information to be publicised even if there is no realistic prospect of any detrimental effects. Consider a thought experiment in which someone plans to divulge some particularly sensitive information – say, a deeply embarrassing fact about you – so it becomes common knowledge, but (as a condition of the thought experiment) doing so will have no adverse consequences at all. You would surely prefer the revelations not to take place, and you may go to some lengths to object to or prevent them, even though there is no prospect of detrimental effects. Apart from being familiar and intuitively plausible, this phenomenon is frequently mentioned in the privacy literature. For example, Rachels (1975: 325) captures it when he says an 'adequate account of privacy should help us to understand . . . why intrusions into things that are "none of your business" are, as such, offensive'. Without labouring a crucial distinction in normative moral theory, this can be referred to as a deontological, as opposed to consequentialist, account of informational privacy, because the concern is about information being made public 'in principle', and not because of adverse consequences.

But this is not a strong objection to the claim that informational privacy concerns are consequentialist. For one thing, the thought experiment is unrealistic precisely because it fails to acknowledge latent consequentialist concerns. Information that has been publicised is at least potentially damaging; conversely, the only way to be certain that information is not damaging is to keep it secret. One is bound to feel insecure and worry about catastrophic effects of the information being made public, whatever the conditions of a thought experiment. So what seems like a deontological grounding is really consequentialist. Someone might object to this claim and insist it really is only 'intrusions into things that are "none of your business" which are, as such, offensive', because they have absolutely no belief that the information will ever be linked to them. But in that case, public health is in a strong position to respond. Public health is not interested in sensitive information for prurient reasons, but in order to produce significant societal benefits, so the value of using the data surely outweighs the feeling of 'offence' or the sense that the information is 'none of your business'.

Relative Importance of Personal Space and Personal Information

The claim is that there are two sorts of privacy interests, in protecting personal space and in controlling personal information, which are grounded in flourishing and consequentialism, respectively. That these sorts of privacy interests are important in these different ways is not to deny that both are important. Nonetheless, the privacy interest in maintaining and protecting personal space is typically more important than the privacy interest in controlling personal information. This has already been hinted at in the way the distinction has been drawn. Presenting personal privacy interests in terms of flourishing suggests that it is always, and always very, important. By contrast, informational privacy interests were explained in consequentialist terms, and divulging information does not necessarily or always have adverse consequences in terms of creating risks and harm. People can acquire even very personal information about others without any bad effects; information can be treated with discrete respect, for example. And even when disclosure does incur risks and harm, these can be minor or mitigated.

The claim that personal privacy is typically more important than informational privacy has to be given some nuance. There is space here for two embellishments. The first involves the 'privacy paradox', encountered in the previous discussion of changing privacy attitudes. To recall, this refers to the disparity between what people say about informational privacy and their actual behaviours regarding their personal information. In particular, it is typical for people to voice anxiety about informational privacy whilst evidently being prepared to generate and share personal information. The privacy paradox is the subject of a sizeable literature, including both explanations of, and scepticism about, the phenomenon. But the point in the present context is that only attitudes towards informational privacy concerns are paradoxical. As Kokolakis (2017), in a very useful summary of the current debate puts it: '*Privacy paradox* is used in this paper as a shortcut for the more accurate term *informational privacy paradox*'. There is no equivalent personal privacy paradox. For example, there is no evidence of a general trend for people to say they are anxious to protect a personal space in which to enjoy solitude or intimacy, on the one hand, whilst behaving in ways which belie this concern on the other. This concurs with the analysis presented here. The need to build personal space into the architecture of our lives is too deep and fundamental to admit of a personal privacy paradox; by contrast, informational privacy interests are malleable and susceptible to sociocultural changes.

The second embellishment is to emphasise that the claim throughout has been that our privacy interest in maintaining and protecting a personal sphere is only typically, and neither universally nor necessarily, more important than our privacy interest in controlling access to and use of personal information. In certain circumstances, the latter matters more than the former. Some incursions into one's personal space are minor, manageable and justified; nothing so grand as one's well-being is at stake. Conversely, informational privacy can be paramount. Information about ethnic identity, for example, has had people incarcerated or killed. Nonetheless, the point stands that personal privacy is typically very important and more important than informational privacy, because of its being required for flourishing, constitutive of well-being and the good life of a human being. Compare other such goods: friendship, for example, is neither universally nor necessarily more important than other goods; but given its constitutive role in the good life, it usually is.

PRIVACY AND PUBLIC HEALTH INFORMATION

The reason for labouring an account of privacy which distinguishes two sorts of privacy interests is that informational, and not personal, privacy concerns are relevant to public health. In other words, public health relies heavily on information, but only very rarely requires incursions into people's personal space.

To illustrate, recall the taxonomy of public health information presented in chapter 1: public health information is collected by research studies, surveillance, data collection during emergencies and service evaluations; sources of information include health activity data, biobanks and novel forms such as the Internet and social media; and this information is used for secondary analysis, data linkage and generating 'big data'. None of these usually requires incursions into people's personal space. This is particularly obvious in some cases; for example, health activity data such as electronic health records, or social media data, already exist, so there can be no question of frustrating the privacy interest in maintaining a private sphere or zone in order to gather it. There are exceptions – data gathering can involve methodologies which threaten personal privacy, such as certain observational studies – but these are rare and require special management.

So, in public health, privacy concerns are about controlling personal information not protecting personal space. This is important in the following way. To recall, personal privacy is typically a very weighty matter, because personal space is required for certain experiences – notably, solitude and intimacy – which are fundamental for flourishing. By contrast, informational privacy is typically (though, as pointed out above, not always) less significant, because some disclosures create no, minimal or manageable risks. The debate about public health information is distorted by a failure to distinguish clearly these two sorts of privacy concerns, because this brings the weightiness of personal privacy interest to bear, when the relevant privacy interest is in the (generally speaking) less weighty matter of controlling personal information. The upshot is that privacy concerns in public health are exaggerated.

A couple of illustrations will clarify the point. In one of a long series of influential publications, Moore (2003) presents an account of the meaning and value of privacy. He succinctly captures the distinction in the dualistic account presented here: 'Privacy, whether physical or informational, is valuable for beings like us' (p. 215). He then does an excellent job of grounding the value of privacy in flourishing and well-being, drawing on the kinds of anthropological and animal studies referred to previously. But throughout, Moore subsumes personal space and informational control under the generic term 'privacy'; as a result, he claims that both sorts of privacy interests – in protecting personal space and controlling personal information – are grounded in flourishing and well-being: 'The ability to regulate access to our bodies, capacities, and powers, as well as sensitive personal information, is an essential part of human flourishing and well-being' (p. 223; see also Moore 2007: 818). But only personal space (and not informational privacy) is so grounded.

Moore is analysing privacy in general, so an even more telling illustration of the same mistake is from the literature on public health information. Take, for example, the following eliding of the distinction between personal and informational privacy concerns by writers on research using biobanked materials for public health purposes:

> The right to privacy is the right to a personal sphere, free from public attention and interference. It includes the right to keep certain facts about oneself secret (Eriksson and Helgesson 2005: 1073).

Subsuming the concern for a personal sphere and secret facts under a generic 'privacy right' has the same effect as Moore's approach, namely, privacy concerns in public health are bound to be overstated, because public health information will inevitably seem seriously problematic when the typically weighty but largely irrelevant matter of protecting personal space – Eriksson and Helgesson's 'personal sphere' – is implicated.

CONCLUDING REMARKS

Maintaining a clear focus on the relevant sort of privacy concern – to control access to and disclosure of one's information – introduces another, less subtle ramification. As laboured in this chapter, privacy concerns about personal information are consequentialist in nature; protecting personal information is important because of the risks of harm created by disclosures. In turn, this suggests a two-fold strategy for meeting privacy concerns in public health, which is pursued in the rest of this book. The first part of the strategy involves identifying harm created by public health information: what sorts of data used in public health create harm, and what sorts of harm do they create? The distinction between anonymous and identifiable data is clearly going to be crucial to this, so these are discussed in the next two chapters, respectively. The second part of the strategy is to devise ways to ameliorate the risks of harm created by public health information. The consent requirement on using personal information, and trust in public health institutions, are important here, so they are discussed in chapters 6 and 7, respectively. The flow of the argument is toward a comprehensive defence of acquiring and using information for public health.

Chapter 4

Anonymity and Reidentification

The previous chapter established that privacy concerns about personal information used in public health are consequentialist; i.e. they centre on the risks of harm created by disclosures. So this chapter examines the harms created by public health data. This cannot be pursued without first analysing 'harm', since this is a contested concept, so the first part of the chapter reviews the harm literature. Since the debate about harm is at an impasse, an inclusive analysis is recommended: 'harm' will be used to refer to any of the conditions in standard accounts. The second part of the chapter addresses the role of anonymity in managing informational harm. Anonymity is central because it is traditionally assumed that anonymous data do not create informational risks. This would be very convenient, because whole swathes of public health information are anonymous. But there is a major challenge to reliance on anonymity in public health from reidentification science, i.e. the increasingly sophisticated ways in which putatively anonymous information can be reidentified. If unmet, the upshot of this challenge is that there are no genuinely anonymous data. So the second half of the chapter meets the challenge to traditional reliance on anonymity in public health presented by reidentification science.

CONCEPTUAL ANALYSIS OF HARM

Public health information is ethically problematic just if its acquisition or use creates serious risks of harm. This claim can be taken in various ways, from being a *prima facie* to a conclusive objection against a piece of public health information. But however it is interpreted, the claim requires an analysis of the central moral concept, harm. In fact, harm is morally important in personal, professional and political life: there is a strong moral prohibition on each of us to avoid harming one another; the Hippocratic Oath requires that physicians 'first do no harm' (*primum non nocere*); and Mill's harm principle relates state interference in a citizen's life to the avoidance of third-part harms. Its significance in various spheres of moral life drives the imperative to understand harm. On the one hand, this has generated a vast literature; on the other, the harm literature has resolved itself into a settled dialectic. The contours of this terrain are so familiar it can be quickly mapped.

Standard Accounts of Harm

Intuitively, one is harmed by being made worse off. For example, you harm someone by punching them on the nose, because they are worse off for being punched. Two things follow from this: harm is a matter of being put in a bad state; and harm is comparative in that it is a matter of being put in a state worse than some other. What other state? Two answers lead to two comparative state-based accounts of harm. The first is the temporal comparative account: you are harmed by being made worse off than you were before the harming event. But there are counterexamples; deliberately denying a patient a painkiller surely harms the patient, but it does not make him or her worse off than he or she was.

This ushers in a second state-based account, the counterfactual comparative account: you are harmed not by being made worse off than you were, but worse off than you would have been without the harming event. This deals with the painkiller case – denying the patient the painkiller does not make him or her worse off than he or she was, it makes them worse off than they would have been had they been given the painkiller – but it is vulnerable to other counterexamples. Suppose someone shoots you, but it so happens that, had the person not, someone else would have; the shooting does not make you worse off than you would have been had the person refrained from shooting you, because the other person would have shot you anyway; but surely the first shooter harms you by shooting you.

The response to these problems retains the intuition that harm is a matter of being put in a bad state, but denies that what makes a state bad is that it is worse than some other state (i.e. the one you were in or could have been in). Rather, some states are just bad in themselves – intrinsically, absolutely or noninstrumentally – and harm is a matter of putting someone in such a state. This requires an account of intrinsically bad states. Oft-cited examples are, 'harm involves conditions that generate a significant chasm or conflict between one's will and one's experience, one's life more broadly understood, or one's circumstances' (Shiffrin 1999: 123), and 'one harms someone if one causes him pain, mental or physical discomfort, disease, deformity, disability, or death' (Harman 2009: 139). There are significant differences between noncomparative bad-state accounts – Harman's is only a sufficient condition, Shiffrin appeals to a disconnection between one's rational will and one's state, for example – but they share the core claim that bad states are bad in themselves and not by comparison with some other state, and they tend to converge on the same kinds of intrinsically bad states, such as those Harman lists.

But they also are all vulnerable to a shared objection. To illustrate, take illness as an example of an intrinsically bad state, such that putting someone in that state harms him or her. We can only get a grip on the bad state of illness by reference to the good state of being healthy. This illness threshold can be disputed, but there must be one. Some people will be above the illness threshold – healthy, not ill – and to varying extents. For example, some will be fit, some super-fit, others super-super-fit. Now suppose someone deliberately impairs a super-super-fit athlete and reduces him or her to being merely super-fit; the person mildly poisons the athlete in some way, for example. Poisoning the athlete is clearly harmful, but not according to the noncomparative bad state account, because the poisoning action does not put the athlete in the intrinsically bad state of illness. Of course, this counterintuitive result is avoided by pointing out that the person made the super-super-fit athlete worse off; but that is to revert back to the comparative bad state account.

The response to these problems is to deny that harm is a matter of being put in a bad state. This is to shift from bad-state to event-based accounts of harm. Hanser (2008) is an exponent, the core elements of his position being as follows. Goods are things that are good to have; basic goods are physical and mental powers or abilities that enable us to achieve a happy life; sight, for example, is a basic good; harm is the event of losing some quantity of a basic good. Hanser embellishes this account in various ways – notably, to incorporate preventive harms and benefits – the details of which need not detain us here. But it is worth clarifying the subtly of his position. Hanser is addressing the question, in virtue of what is a harm; and his answer is, in virtue of its being the loss of a basic good. So a harm is a harm independently of the badness of the resultant state of the harmed individual; hence, one is harmed by the loss of a basic good even if ultimately one ends up in a better state than before the harm:

> But according to the account I have proposed, the badness of lacking a basic good does not explain why losing it constitutes a harm. Losing a basic good constitutes a harm simply because it is the losing of a good. The event is bad in its own right, so to speak, quite independently of the badness of its end-state (Hanser 2008: 443–444).

In light of this, some objections miss the mark. In particular, some critics object that 'loss' is a comparative notion, so Hanser's event-based account is bound to collapse into a comparative account. For instance, to lose a basic good is to go from having it at one time to not having it at a later time, and this is just the temporal comparative account again (*mutatis mutandis* for preventive harms; see Klocksiem 2012: 288). This misses the mark because, on the temporal comparative account, what makes the harm a harm is the relative badness of the relevant states – so the action ceases to be a harm if the latter state is no worse than the preceding state – whereas on the event-based account, what makes the harm a harm is the loss of a basic good, so it remains harmful whatever the harmed individual's final state.

But event-based accounts are vulnerable to other objections. Hanser's, for example, is a biconditional account: one suffers a harm if and only if one loses some quantity of a basic good. In other words, losing some quantity of a basic good is sufficient and necessary for harm. But there are counterexamples. To illustrate, consider the necessity claim that one suffers harm only if one loses some quantity of a basic good. A basic good is some mental or physical ability or power which enables one to live a happy life. Now suppose someone deliberately puts you in pain. He harms you, but you do not lose any quantity of a basic good. A possible reply is that being pain-free is required to live a happy life; but whilst that is true, being pain-free is not an ability or power of the sort Hanser means by a basic good (Bradley 2012: 404). This is not just a technical objection to event-based accounts; rather, it captures an intuitive problem, because what really motivates us to say that someone has harmed you is simply that he put you in pain, which is an intrinsically bad state. This is just the noncomparative bad-state account again. So whilst Hanser's event-based account might well capture something of what we mean by harm – usually, the loss of a basic good is harmful – it does not capture well all of what we ordinarily mean by harm.

Impasse

By now, a familiar dialectical structure has emerged. We are trying to understand harm, as a precursor to evaluating harm created by public health information. An analysis is proposed. Objections are presented, usually appealing to counterexamples. So an alternative analysis is proposed. Further objections are presented, appealing to different counterexamples. So a further alternative analysis is proposed. And so on. The upshot is an impasse. A couple of features of this literary terrain are worth pointing out because they elucidate the impasse.

It is typical for writers on harm to list desiderata and puzzling cases, then advocate their preferred analysis by showing how it meets these or, at least, meets them better than do rival accounts (Hanser 2008: 427–440, 445–449; Klocksiem 2012: 285–287, 290–296; Bradley 2012: 394–396). There is considerable overlap between lists of desiderata and puzzling cases. For example, most people think unity is desirable – i.e. an account should identify the core of harm which explains all cases – and cite Parfit's nonidentity problem and death as difficult cases a successful account of harm should be able to handle. Some accounts of harm are a direct response to a specific desideratum or puzzling case; for example, Bradley (2012: 398) says that Harman 'is concerned about the implications of the comparative account in non-identity cases'. But surely it is highly implausible that any one account of harm will satisfy a list of desiderata and deal with a number of very puzzling cases. More likely, an account will score well in some respects – meet the unity criterion, explain how death is a harm or whatever – but not all. Hence the dialectical structure and inevitable impasse previously sketched.

When a conceptual analysis reaches this sort of impasse, there are numerous typical responses, all of which figure in the harm literature. One move is to vigorously defend one of the proposed analyses. Klocksiem (2012), for example, is an 'attempt to show that none of the objections to the counterfactual account are ultimately successful'. These always generate interesting insights, but are destined to fail; how likely is it that any of the standard analyses of harm will, after all, turn out to be correct and command a consensus? Another move is to add to the inventory of available accounts in the hope of finally defining harm. Although such innovations are disparate, they share the same problem. Basically, innovative additions to the inventory of accounts of harm face a dilemma between being plausible and substantive. In other words, the new account might seem plausible, but only because it collapses into some other familiar account; or it remains distinct, in which case the plausibility dissipates. There is room here for one case in point.

Petersen (2014) suggests a third version of the comparative bad-state account to add to the temporal and counterfactual accounts: harm is a matter of lowering someone's level of well-being to below the 'well-being for mankind' (see also Dare 1998; Harrosh 2012). But the baseline account faces the dilemma just outlined between being plausible and substantive. On the one hand, any plausibility is due to its being a mishmash of the temporal and counterfactual accounts, i.e. taking someone below the 'well-being for mankind' makes them worse off than they were and/or worse off than they could have been. On the other hand, as a distinctive account it is highly implausible: what is this 'baseline' one is harmed by being taken below? In particular, '[hu]mankind' does not have a baseline; rather there is massive cultural, social, etc. variation between welfare baselines, so how can this be a unified account of harm? In sum, innovations delay as opposed to avoid the impasse about harm.

Given this impasse, it is unsurprising that some writers advocate eliminativism about harm:

> Unfortunately, when we look at attempts to explain the nature of harm, we find a mess. The most widely discussed account, the comparative account, faces counterexamples that seem fatal. But no alternative account has gained any currency [. . .] isn't it possible that a plausible account will be forthcoming? . . . I will discuss reasons to think that the answer is no (Bradley (2012: 391).

On this basis, Bradley suggests we 'avoid appealing to the notion of harm at all in our moral theorizing...Let harm go the way of phlogiston' (pp. 410–411). But this is surely to be avoided, because eliminating harm as a substantive concept would be counterintuitive and compromise moral theorizing.

An Inclusive Account of Harm

We need to navigate a way through this impasse in order to get onto the main business of evaluating harm created by public health information. The best response to the impasse is to advocate not one but many of the accounts of harm: 'I suspect that a pluralist or disjunctive account of harm, which includes both comparative and noncomparative dimensions, is unavoidable' (McMahan 2013: 8). Pluralism is the view that a full analysis of harm will involve many features of the main rival accounts; disjunctivism is the view that to harm someone is to make him or her worse off or put him or her in an intrinsically bad state (or some other account). This approach has been developed elsewhere, albeit in somewhat disparate ways. For example, Woollard (2012: 689) astutely observes that 'we are pulled between these two ways of understanding harming [non-comparative and overall-comparison harming] . . . both types of harming are morally relevant', though she goes on to suggest that the significance of noncomparative harm is relatively limited. And Meyer (2016: S.3.4) illustrates the obvious advantage of disjunctive accounts, namely, that counterexamples to one account can be handled by an appeal to the other.

This inclusive approach will be taken here. It is useful for 'harm' to continue to figure in the discussion as a heuristic device. Although none of the accounts of harm canvassed in this section is fully convincing, each captures something of the way we use the ordinary word 'harm' to refer to a disvalue. So we should make expansive use of the term, taking 'harm' to include making someone worse off than he or she was or would have been otherwise (in either a physical or moral sense), or putting someone in an obviously bad state (in pain, for example), or reducing the powers or abilities required for someone to lead a happy life (such as eyesight) or any other plausible account of harm. Any such action is clearly *prima facie* questionable and in need of justification, whether or not any one of them is the correct definition of 'harm'. This approach does not rule out informational harm by definition or stipulation; in fact, it puts the dialectical onus on the defence of public health information in this book, because no sort of harm has been conceptually rejected, so all the detrimental effects of gathering and using data are relevant. So we can proceed to ask whether, in what ways, and to what extent public health information harms people, in any sense; and, if it does, whether it is nonetheless justified by its societal benefits.

ANONYMITY AND THE CHALLENGE OF REIDENTIFICATION

In managing informational harm, anonymity is crucial. Information does not seem to create any risk of harm if it cannot be ascribed to anyone, so anonymous information seems unobjectionable. Hence, 'the foundation of much privacy regulation is that if there is no personally identifiable information, there is no privacy harm' (Kaplan 2015: 259). In turn, studies involving anonymous information do not require stringent governance; in particular, ethics committees either waive approval or require only a light review. By contrast, information which is attributable to an individual is a potential source of harm, so requires more ethical and governance oversight.

This is the basis of an established 'binary model' for managing informational risk, in which there are two categories of data: anonymous information which 'does not sacrifice individual privacy' (Bernheim et al. 2013: 39) versus other, potentially harmful data. Though the subject of query and controversy – the *Source Informatics* and *Sorrell* cases in the UK and US, respectively, in which companies requested to purchase anonymous prescribing data, are well-documented examples (Dunkel 2001; Kaplan 2015) – the binary model, and its reliance on anonymity, have been fundamental to the general management of informational risks and protection of informational privacy.

More to the point, anonymity is particularly important in public health. Of course, public health cannot rely solely on anonymous data, but also requires identifiable data, which we turn to in the next chapter. Nonetheless, public health addresses population level issues – protecting and promoting the health of populations – so many public health goals can be achieved using large, aggregated, anonymous data sets. To refer back to the taxonomy of public health information in chapter 1, monitoring the prevalence of diseases for surveillance purposes, data on service uptake for service evaluations, secondary uses of data to identify public health risks, and so on, require only anonymous and not identifiable information. On the binary model, such information is ethically unproblematic so escapes privacy regulation and does not require close ethical scrutiny or stringent governance. In particular, ethics committees typically either do not need to approve the collection, use and sharing of anonymous public health information or, if they do, require only a light-touch review.

Some Initial Objections to Reliance on Anonymity

This assumption that anonymous information does not create risks of harm can be queried. For one thing, individuals might object that 'intrusions into things that are "none of your business" are, as such, offensive' (Rachels 1975: 325), even if the relevant information is anonymous. This was dealt with in the discussion of whether privacy concerns are deontic in chapter 3. If the 'offence' is based on the consequentialist concern that the only way to be certain that one's information will remain anonymous is to refuse to disclose it in the first place, it is best deferred until the forthcoming discussion of reidentification. If the 'offence' is based on the deontological principle that it is wrong in itself to acquire and use one's anonymised sensitive data, it is overridden by the societal benefits of public health information.

Another counterargument centring on the individual is that one's anonymous data might be used for purposes considered repugnant, such as research in assisted reproduction or embryology, on animals, or to increase the profits of dubious commercial interests (Kaplan 2015: 259). But the real issue here is consent to uses of one's data, so it is best deferred until the discussion of consent in chapter 6. The other sort of counterargument to the claim that anonymous information does not create any risk of harm centres not on individuals, but on groups or societies to which they belong. In particular, anonymous data might further stigmatize disadvantaged social groups. This is important, but it belongs in an analysis of the harm of stigmatization created by public health information, which will be discussed in the next chapter.

Reidentification Science

We can pursue the present argument on the basis that anonymous information is unobjectionable, and does not require close ethical scrutiny or stringent governance. But there is an important challenge to this seemingly happy outcome. To explain the challenge requires clarifying distinctions that have so far been elided.

There are three sorts of data, traditionally defined as follows. Identified information is information which is linked to an individual. Anonymous information is information which cannot be linked to an individual. In between these is 'de-identified' data, where de-identification 'is the act of reducing the information content in data to decrease the probability of discovering an individual's identity' (El Emam et al. 2011). There are myriad complications around this tripartite distinction. The terminology is messy, with key terms, such as 'personal data' and 'anonymization' being defined and used interchangeably and differently; and there are various de-identification techniques, some of which are well-established (aggregation, data masking and so on), others more innovative (Gkoulalas-Divanis and Loukides 2015). Attempts to interpret the recent European Union's General Data Protection Regulation (GDPR) is a good illustration. Recital 26 explicitly states that the GDPR 'do[es] not apply to anonymous information, namely information which does not relate to an identified or identifiable natural person or to personal data rendered anonymous in such a manner that the data subject is not or no longer identifiable'. So the GDPR operates on the binary model. But in the regulations, 'personal data' is defined as 'any information relating to an identified or identifiable natural person', and this includes 'pseudonymised data':

> 'Pseudonymisation' means the processing of personal data in such a manner that the personal data can no longer be attributed to a specific data subject without the use of additional information, provided that such additional information is kept separately and is subject to technical and organisational measures to ensure that the personal data are not attributed to an identified or identifiable natural person (Article 4[5] GDPR).

This might seem straightforward, but the GDPR definition of 'pseudonymisation' is crucially different to conventional definitions and, arguably, allows for some pseudonymised data to be personal whilst others are anonymous (Mourby et al. 2018). We return to the GDPR case later in this discussion, but these complications need not detain us here, because the tripartite distinction, and the challenge to public health's reliance on the binary model which emanates from it, are clear enough.

The crucial point is that the middle category of de-identified (or anonymised or pseudonymised) information is reidentifiable. In other words, although data are rendered anonymous, it is possible to relink the information to an individual. For example, anyone with the relevant key or code can reidentify pseudonymised data. Worries about anonymity are at least as old as the Internet (Froomkin 1995), and the mere possibility of reidentifying de-identified data might not seem particularly challenging. But advances in 're-identification science' have created ever more sophisticated ways of reidentifying putatively anonymised data. This is facilitated by features of the 'digital age', notably the massive proliferation of personal information and increasingly powerful computers and data mining techniques. As a result, re-identification 'attacks' by 'adversaries' have achieved striking, notorious, well-documented successes (Ohm 2010: 1716–1723).

The development and success of reidentification science seems to require that we replace distinctions between sorts of data – some of which are considered to be ethically unproblematic – with a continuum or spectrum of information:

> Most privacy laws treat the identifiability of information as a binary construct: information is either identifiable (personal) or not. In reality, however, a continuum of identifiability exists, with some data sets being quite easy to re-identify with minimal resources and skill, and others requiring considerable time, effort, cost, and skill to re-identify (El Emam 2010: 64).

In other words, there are no longer differences in kind between data – anonymous versus identifiable, for example – only differences in the degree of difficulty or likelihood of, or potential for, reidentification (McGrail, Gutteridge and Meagher 2015; Nuffield Council on Bioethics 2015: 66–72).

Evidently, this undermines reliance in data management on the tripartite distinction between identified, de-identified and anonymous information, and the binary model in which anonymous data are ethically unproblematic. More specifically, it presents a significant challenge for public health, because, as outlined, anonymity is particularly crucial to the justification for gathering and using public health information. So in order to defend public health information, this challenge has to be met.

Responses to the Reidentification Challenge

One strategy is to query the claims made for reidentification science (Cavoukian and El Emam 2011; Cavoukian and Castro 2014). A version of this is to refine de-identification techniques until at least some data are immune from reidentification (Gkoulalas-Divanis and Loukides 2015). But to meet the challenge of reidentification on technical grounds is bound to be unsatisfactory. For one thing, there is a trade-off between privacy protection and data quality. Ensuring anonymity by utilising de-identification techniques that render the data useless for public health purposes would be a pyrrhic victory: 'secure de-identification of rich data is probably not possible without substantially degrading the data' (Culnane, Rubinstein and Teague 2017). Besides, the discussion would collapse into a dispute between computer scientists, which would not only be arcane, it would remain unsettled, because information technology is constantly and rapidly developing. More important, the view that reidentification remains a serious challenge to reliance on anonymity in data management would win out – no matter how much we improve de-identification techniques – by appeal to the inductive argument that we can infer from previous unanticipated successes in reidentifying data that the science will develop.

Given that we cannot rely on purely technical responses to the reidentification challenge (though of course the risk of the reidentification can be reduced by refining de-identification techniques) we should treat all data as more or less reidentifiable. So the research question is whether we can retain the benefits of the binary model – in which anonymous data were considered unobjectionable and therefore did not require restrictive ethical and governance oversight – despite the power of reidentification science. It will be argued here that we can.

Reidentification Risk

To begin the argument, contrast two seemingly disparate responses to the reidentification challenge. Ohm (2010) describes reliance on anonymity in data management and illustrates the power of reidentification science. He argues on this basis that regulating data by categorising information – anonymous data are ethically and legally unproblematic, for example – is no longer tenable, so recommends abandoning de-identification or anonymization in data management. Ohm then canvasses three responses to this situation – namely, to punish reidentifiers more strictly, rely on a technological breakthrough in anonymization techniques, and ban reidentification – but sees all three as insufficient. Instead, he recommends, 'regulators must ask a broader set of questions that help reveal the risk of reidentification and threat of harm' (p. 1761). In other words, instead of categorising data as anonymous, anonymised or identified, we should undertake an assessment of the risk of reidentification and regulate accordingly.

Schwartz and Solove's (2011) argument shares exactly the same premises as Ohm's (2010): established privacy regulation is based on categorising data – as personally identifiable, and therefore potentially harmful, or not – and this is no longer tenable because 'technologists can take information that appears on its face to be non-identifiable and turn it into identifiable data' (p. 1816). But Schwartz and Solove's argument then takes a quite different turn. Rather than 'abandon' the established approach, as Ohm advocated, Schwartz and Solove recommend retaining and revising the basic structure of the binary model. In particular, the concept of 'personally identifiable information' should be revised to include two sorts of information, namely, 'identified' and 'identifiable' data.

This looks like we are back to categorising data, but Schwartz and Solove suggest that their 'model places information on a continuum that begins with no risk of identification at one end, and ends with identified individuals at the other' (p. 1877). In other words, instead of relying on the old concept of 'personally identifiable information', we should undertake an assessment of the risk of reidentification and regulate accordingly.

Evidently, the dispute between Ohm (2010) and Schwartz and Solove (2011) is not deep (certainly not as deep as the latter suggest: see pp. 1865ff). Their substantive views are identical: both Ohm, and Schwartz and Solove, conclude that, given the already high and ever-increasing threat to de-identification, the key to data management is an assessment of the risk of reidentification. In fact, their dispute is merely verbal. As Ohm (2010: 1744) puts it:

> We are using the wrong terms, and we need to stop. We must abolish the word anonymize; let us simply strike it from our debates. A word that should mean, "try to achieve anonymity" is too often understood to mean "achieve anonymity".

By contrast, Schwartz and Solove (2011: 1865) say:

> Existing definitions of [personally identifiable information] have proven problematic. Nonetheless, we reject the idea that privacy law should abandon the concept.

As these comments indicate – and since their respective arguments culminate in the same basis for data regulation, namely, an assessment of risk of reidentification – their dispute is over nothing more substantive than whether to retain words such as 'anonymize' and how to define the concept of 'personally identifiable information'.

The point of this analysis of Ohm (2010) and Schwartz and Solove (2011) is that seemingly disparate – even seemingly adversarial – responses to the reidentification challenge to anonymity collapse into the same substantive view, namely, that data management should be based on an assessment of the risks of reidentification. This conclusion does not just apply to these papers, but can be generalised. After all, there are only two sorts of responses to the reidentification challenge – either abandon or revise our current reliance on categorising data as anonymous – and these responses have been represented by Ohm (2010) and Schwartz and Solove (2011), respectively. So we have exhausted all the options; and, as the analysis suggests, they collapse into the same strategy of regulating information by assessing the risk of reidentification. A response to this is that there could be other versions of each strategy: one might agree with Ohm and 'abandon anonymization', or with Schwartz and Solove and 'revise personally identifiable information', but suggest some alternative other than 'assess the risk of reidentification'. But what would this be? If the challenge is that of reidentification, it is obvious that data regulation will have to be based on an assessment of the risks of reidentification. Hence, such seemingly disparate arguments as Ohm's and Schwartz and Solove's, were bound to collapse into one another.

Risk of Reindentifying Public Health Information

The upshot of this discussion is a strategy for meeting the reidentification challenge to relying on anonymity in public health: determine the likelihood that public health information will be reidentified. It is argued here that the current risk of reidentifying public health data is already low and can be made even lower.

In developing this, Ohm (2010) is again informative, because he suggests five 'factors to determine the risk of reidentification' (pp. 1764 ff): data-handling techniques, private versus public data release, quantity of data collected and retained, motive to reidentify, and trust in people or institutions. These are ambiguous between being factors in assessing versus reducing reidentification risk – Ohm presents them as the former, but uses them in illustrations of how the current level of reidentification risk can be reduced – but we can take them as both. Furthermore, Ohm presents this five-fold list as neither definitive nor exhaustive; he contrasts his list with that of the 'European privacy watchdog, the Article 29 Working Group' (p. 1764), and he suggests important additional considerations, namely, sensitivity of, and potential benefits from, data (p. 1768).

Ohm then uses these factors to assess the risk of the reidentification of health information (pp. 1769–1771). Health information, being both highly sensitive and beneficial, creates a particularly acute dilemma between privacy and utility which can no longer be navigated by relying on anonymization. Rather, we should focus on trust; erstwhile 'informal rules and soft intuitions…must be formalised and codified', and this can be backed up, for example, by new sanctions, mandated technological mechanisms and additional protections for more sensitive data. As this suggests, Ohm's assessment of the risk of reidentification does not promote restriction of health information. On the contrary, the most striking part of Ohm's assessment is that 'abandoning anonymization' and relying instead on factors such as trust will increase the amount of health information:

> Researchers who share data according to the new trust-based guidelines will be permitted to share *all* data, even fields of data like birth date or full ZIP code that they cannot access today. With more data and more specific data, researchers will be able to produce more accurate results, and thereby hopefully come to quicker and better conclusions [. . .] Researchers should be allowed to release full, unscrubbed databases to verifiably trusted third parties, subject to new controls on use and new penalties for abuse (Ohm 2010: 1771).

One set of researchers who stand to benefit is epidemiologists, whose access to information has been made harder by restrictions, without commensurable increases in privacy (n.315). So, according to Ohm's assessment, public health can have the benefits of anonymity – collection, use and flow of health information – whilst fully recognising the power of reidentification science.

Further Risk-Reducing Strategies

We can go further. Ohm focused on one of his five factors, trust, and this is endorsed (and augmented) in the discussion of public trust in chapter 7. The point to note here is that all four of his other factors apply more than his discussion might suggest. To illustrate, it is useful to distinguish two sorts of 'adversaries' (the term used in this literature for reidentifiers of data): adversaries from within public health, and external adversaries (cf. Benitez and Malin 2010).

To take each in turn, how likely is it that public health adversaries will reidentify data? Motive seems particularly relevant here. As mentioned a number of times, public health goals to which information is important – protecting and promoting population health – can be achieved without identifying data. This indicates that there is little motivation from within public health to reidentify. Ohm is alert to this, pointing out that 'rules governing what academic researchers can do with data should reflect the fact that academic researchers rarely desire to reidentify people in their datasets', and taking 'health privacy' as a case in point. Not only is there little incentive for public health professionals and institutions to reidentify data, there is a massive disincentive. Public health is not a resource-rich field. On the contrary, it is highly implausible that individuals or institutions in public health have the time or money to bother reidentifying information. So, there is little incentive, and serious disincentive, for public health adversaries to reidentify data.

External adversaries might seem more threatening. But as Ohm suggests, regulators should 'weigh economic incentives for reidentification', approving of Cline's (2009) point that there is 'far less economic incentive for a criminal to go after medical data instead of credit card information . . . If *I'm* a criminal with advanced data skills and I have a day to spend, I'm going to go after financial data and not health data'. This seems right: an external adversary's main targets will be directly financial (or indirectly financial in some form of surveillance capitalism) – or based on some other clear motive, such as revealing and influencing voting patterns – as opposed to being health related. Furthermore, we can appeal to Ohm's other 'factors'. His distinction between public and private release of information seems relevant, for example. As frequently mentioned, and as Ohm points out, eye-catching reidentification requires publicly available data sets, but public health does not require the public release of information.

A case in point is Hauge et al.'s (2016) application of geographical profiling techniques to identify the pseudonymous British artist 'Banksy'. In an 'Ethical note', Hauge et al. explicitly defend their study by pointing out that they 'only used data in the public domain' (p. 189). Whatever the ethical merits of this defence, the study simply could not have been undertaken had the relevant data not been publicly accessible. Likewise, the threat of reidentifying public health information is at least significantly reduced by keeping it out of the public domain. This is not to deny that public health requires dissemination, but not of raw data; we need to publicise broad epidemiological trends, links between lifestyle choices and health risks, and so on, not the data sets on which such findings are based.

The argument presented here can be framed by reference to the GDPR. As mentioned above, the GDPR seems to suggest that data which have undergone a process of 'pseudonymisation' should be treated as personal data. But GDPR, Recital 26 clearly states that the status of pseudonymised data is moot:

> To determine whether a natural person is identifiable, account should be taken of all the means reasonably likely to be used, such as singling out, either by the controller or by another person to identify the natural person directly or indirectly. To ascertain whether means are reasonably likely to be used to identify the natural person, account should be taken of all objective factors, such as the costs of and the amount of time required for identification, taking into consideration the available technology at the time of the processing and technological developments.

In effect, the argument presented in this section is that when 'objective factors' – Recital 26 mentions costs, time required, available technology – are taken into account, reidentification of standard public health information by adversaries within or external to public health is not 'reasonably likely'.

Reviews of evidence of reidentification attacks on health data support the argument presented here. The claim that the risk of reidentification of public health data is already low, and can be even further reduced, is confirmed by El Emam et al. (2011), who point out that, whilst the notorious reidentification attacks mentioned seem to demonstrate 'a failure of de-identification . . . there has been no formal investigation to assess this evidence, and in particular, to contrast the reidentification attacks on health data with other types of data'. To address this, El Emam et al. undertook a systematic review. Particularly notable findings include: few of the reidentification attacks were on health data; most were undertaken by researchers to expose, not exploit, the risk of reidentification; and the vast majority of data that were reidentified had not been properly de-identified.

El Emam et al.'s analysis supports the view that the risk of health data reidentification is lower than might be inferred by notorious reidentification attacks, and can be made lower by, for example, de-identifying data properly. And this has been subsequently reconfirmed by more recent evaluations of the risk of reidentification of health data, and technical solutions for reducing reidentification risk (Joly et al. 2015; Salloway 2016; cf. Hansson et al. 2016: 1555).

OBJECTIONS

There is space to consider some objections to the argument presented in the previous section. One response to the argument might be that it is dangerously incautious; another is that it might have longer term or indirect consequences. In this section, versions of each of these responses are considered in turn.

Precautionary Principle

A possible objection to the argument presented here appeals to the precautionary principle. As is well documented, the principle is vexed, because there is no consensus on its definition, and it seems to suffer from the fatal flaw that neither the strong nor weak version is tenable (Steel 2015). We do not need to go deeply into this controversy; the basic idea is plausible and influential. Policy ought to be based on scientific evidence. But sometimes policy decisions have to be made in unusual circumstances: foreseeable serious risk, but considerable scientific uncertainty. The gist of the principle is that, in such circumstances, the evidential bar on policy should be lowered, and we should implement preventive policies to avoid risks, despite less scientific evidence than we usually demand. The principle was developed in the context of environmental policy (Stewart 2002), and the classic application is to climate change: there are foreseeable risks; the scientific evidence is incomplete and contested; nonetheless, we ought to implement climate change policies to prevent the catastrophic effects of global warming.

The same line of thought has been applied to data management in light of the reidentification challenge. For example, Narayanan, Huey and Felten (2016) show that there is evidence of risk ('Significant privacy risks stem from current de-identification practices') in the context of scientific uncertainty ('the chances of reidentification depend highly on the progress of reidentification tools and the auxiliary datasets available to an adversary [so] probability of a privacy violation in the future is essentially unknowable'). Their response is a 'weak version of the precautionary approach' (pp. 357–358), resulting in various data policy recommendations. Their detailed proposal is not so important, because they are focused on public release of ad hoc de-identified data, and this is hardly standard public health practice. The general point is that reidentification is both risky and uncertain, so we should abide by the precautionary principle, and this means increased data restrictions. Applied specifically to public health, the upshot would be more restrictive public health data management on precautionary grounds.

But restricting public health information by appeal to the precautionary principle is not compelling. The basic problem is that there are two sets of foreseeable risks which arise in conditions of scientific uncertainty, and the precautionary principle can be invoked in response to either of them. The first is risk of privacy harms from reidentification; as noted, Narayanan, Huey and Felten (2016) invoked the precautionary principle to justify data restrictions to avoid these. But the second set of risks are health threats which public health is designed to prevent, such as disease outbreaks. The most familiar application of the precautionary principle in public health ethics is to avoid this second set of risks. For example, 'the precautionary principle has implicitly guided public health interventions designed to limit or forestall epidemic outbreaks' (Bayer and Fairchild 2004: 490; see Holland 2015: 41–43). This clearly extends to information-gathering 'interventions', such as surveillance and data collection during outbreaks.

Invoking the precautionary principle to avoid this second set of risks would justify expansive, as opposed to restrictive, data policy, which is exactly the opposite conclusion to that reached by Narayanan, Huey and Felten (2016). In sum, the precautionary principle cuts both ways: it can be invoked to justify either restrictive or expansive public health data management, depending on which set of risks one is trying to avoid. Since it does not adjudicate between these data policy options, the principle cannot be the basis of an objection to the line of argument in this chapter.

Slippery Slopes

Another possible objection to the argument presented here is a slippery slope objection. The basic form of slippery slope arguments is simple: the action in question is permissible in itself but objectionable because it is at the top of a slippery slope to impermissible actions. The simplicity is deceptive because there are different sorts of slippery slopes (Lamb 2013). The main contrast is between logical and empirical (or psychological) slopes. Logical slopes are slippery because there is no relevant dissimilarity between the permissible action at the top and the impermissible actions at the bottom; so reasons for accepting the former are reasons for accepting the latter; so accepting the former logically commits one to the latter. By contrast, empirical (or psychological) slopes are slippery not because of logical entailment, but because, as a matter of empirical psychological fact, people will go from the permissible action at the top to accepting impermissible actions at the bottom.

The reidentification challenge can be read as a slippery slope argument. Data are not on a continuum or spectrum, but on a slippery slope, from low to high risk of reidentification. So even public health information of low risk of reidentification is objectionable because it is at the top of a slippery slope to public health information at high risk of reidentification. For example, allowing surveillance data, properly de-identified medical records, securely stored biobanked materials and so on is fine, but it is the top of a slippery slope to highly sensitive personal data at much greater risk of a reidentification attack. There is something in this, but it has to be teased out carefully.

First, which sort of slippery slope argument is this, empirical (or psychological) or logical? Arguably, not logical. Degree of risk is usually taken to be a relevant dissimilarity between actions which impacts on practical reasoning. Cycling without a helmet on a quiet country lane is not at the top of a slippery slope to cycling without a helmet on a busy road, because the disparate risk is a relevant dissimilarity, so the former does not logically entail the latter.

A complication here is that there are different versions of logical slippery slopes. One is as follows. There is relevant dissimilarity between the permissible action at the top (call it A) and the impermissible action at the bottom (call it E) of the slippery slope. So there is no direct logical entailment from one to the other. But there are intermediate actions – B, C, D – and no relevant dissimilarities between each of these. So, there is indirect logical entailment from A to E (via B, C, D). Applied to our topic: there is a series of steps from collecting public health data at low risk of reidentification to collecting data at high risk of reidentification. But this is not compelling. The argument would be trading on vagueness; i.e. there is no bright line between data at low versus high risk of reidentification, as the one shades into the other. This is true, but we can still see the logical difference between data on either side of the grey area, just as we can see a reason to wear a helmet while riding a bike on a busy road that does not apply to quiet roads, even though there is no bright line between cycle rides of low and high risk.

So the putative slippery slope from low to high risk of data reidentification must be empirical (or psychological). This is much more plausible. In particular – and to revisit the distinction between adversaries made earlier – it sounds plausible that adversaries from within public health will be disposed to slide down the slope from collecting data of low to high risk of reidentification. It is easy to imagine individuals and institutions becoming complacent about reidentification risks and tempted to gather and use more and more information to achieve public health goals.

Notwithstanding the plausibility, this is not a major objection to the argument of this chapter; rather, it is one of the many points at which to reiterate that this book is not arguing for complacency about data privacy. Of course, public health information can create serious privacy harm to which we must be alert. Sliding down an empirical (or psychological) slippery slope to collecting data at high risk of reidentification is just one case in point. But the best response is to acknowledge the slope, be vigilant about sliding down it and take appropriate preventive measures; not to restrict reliance on public data at low risk of reidentification.

CONCLUDING REMARKS

This chapter has argued that the benefits of the binary model for managing informational risk can be retained despite the reidentification challenge. This is not to downplay the challenge; nonetheless, that the level of current risk is low, and given the variety of ways of reducing it still further, the current and foreseeable risk of reidentification of public health data should be tolerated. After all: 'Anonymisation methods cannot ensure that the risk of reidentification is zero, but this is not the threshold that is expected by privacy laws and regulations in any jurisdiction' (El Emam, Rodgers and Malin 2015: 1). Nor is it expected by the general public, as indicated by studies eliciting people's attitudes to providing their personal health data for public health purposes. For example, Schleidgen et al. (2019) showed that people are prepared to participate in research because they recognise how beneficial it is to public health, even though they perceive a greater than minimal risk of reidentification of their data. So, we ought to accept some risk of reidentification of health information – and more than we would in other informational domains – for the sake of huge societal benefits on offer.

Chapter 5

Identifiable Data

The previous chapter defended reliance on anonymity in managing public health information. But public health cannot rely solely on anonymous information. For one thing, identifiable information is required to achieve vital public health goals. These include epidemiological surveillance, cancer and other disease registries, and secondary purposes, such as audit and service planning, along with data linkage and the ability to follow up individuals (Al-Shahi and Warlow 2000; Black 2003; Souhami 2006; Hansson et al. 2016). In fact, anonymisation can compromise information-gathering activities: 'While protecting privacy, [anonymisation] also eliminates (or at least diminishes) some research possibilities, for example research on often neglected minority groups, individuals with rare diseases, or individuals who live in remote locations' (McGrail, Gutteridge and Meagher 2015: 741). So this chapter addresses the privacy-utility dilemma in the context of identifiable public health information.

In keeping with the overall aim of this book, this chapter defends the use of identifiable public health information. The argument is in three parts. The first section describes the standard way of trading off privacy concerns about, and the social utility of, identifiable public health data, and considers some innovations. The second section takes a novel approach: are there any pervasive influences in the way this trade-off is standardly made? It is argued that the risks and harms said to be created by identifiable public health information are systematically overstated in a number of subtle ways. This has the effect of weighing privacy concerns and claims more heavily than is justified in the trade-off with social utility. The third section takes a different harm-based approach to present a positive argument in favour of using identifiable data in public health. Mill's harm principle is often invoked in public health ethics, but applications of the principle in the context of information gathering and use are limited to communicable disease reporting. It is argued that the principle can justify a greater range of uses of identifiable public health data.

IDENTIFIABLE PUBLIC HEALTH INFORMATION

Identifiable data create the familiar dilemma between, on the one hand, privacy concerns and risks of harm, and, on the other, social utility or public value. The dilemma motivates a debate which has well-documented features. Risks of privacy harm and potential social utility are clarified. Each is weighed, and the trade-off between them negotiated. This usually includes identifying particularly sensitive categories of public health information; genetic data, HIV status and mental health diagnoses are prominent examples. In turn, the sorts of risks and harms created by sensitive data are identified. These typically include stigmatization and discrimination which compromise financial, insurance or employment opportunities. Institutional structures for privacy protection – legal, regulatory and governance systems – are described, critiqued and iteratively developed in light of this privacy-utility trade-off.

A Rawlsian Approach

The debate just outlined is so familiar that one might wonder whether there is more to say about it other than that it is ongoing and important. One way to spice things up is to look at some innovations as to how to prosecute the debate. For example, Moore (2010: 237) establishes a presumption in favour of privacy, but recognises that this can be overridden, so discusses three contrasting cases, namely, the Orchomenos sickle cell anemia case, sexually transmitted disease (STD) and influenza transmission. Moore's discussion illustrates familiar privacy-utility debates, but he goes on to suggest: 'In determining the correct balance between public health and informational privacy John Rawls's notion of placing individuals behind a veil of ignorance may be of some service' (p. 237). Might this appeal to Rawls introduce some innovative ways of trading off privacy and utility in the context of identifiable public health information?

Rawls (1971) presented an entire theory of justice we do not need to go into deeply here; the part relevant to Moore's suggestion is a well-known thought experiment. In choosing principles of justice (Rawls's concern) or how to trade-off informational privacy and public health (our concern) you should place yourself under a veil of ignorance: i.e. you do not know what position you occupy in society. Specifically, you do not know your idiosyncratic characteristics – race, sex, profession, religion, talents, values and so on – including, as Moore points out, whether you are 'a public health official, an infected individual, or someone at risk of being infected'. The idea is that a blind choice will force you to choose fairly, since you do not know in advance how your decision will affect you.

This is an interesting innovation, but its limitations are indicated by Moore's subsequent comments. Moore goes on to illustrate results of the thought experiment: privacy might 'trump public health', or vice versa; or we might reach a compromise between the two. This is all perfectly plausible, but it is unclear that Rawls's 'veil of ignorance' thought experiment is doing any work. To refer to Moore's examples, we do not need Rawls to see that we should not publicise which children have lice, but should publicise information about someone knowingly infecting others with a dangerous disease; and we should not disclose that a person has an STD beyond what is necessary for containment, but should restrict the movements of recalcitrant tuberculosis (TB) carriers (pp. 237–238). We would arrive at these sensible judgements simply by undertaking the trade-off between privacy and utility, familiar from the main body of Moore's paper.

The basic flaw in Moore's suggestion is a category error. It confuses the search for principles (of justice, in Rawls's original presentation) with a decision about whether to side with privacy or utility in specific cases (children with lice, recalcitrant TB carriers and so on). Rawls introduced the veil of ignorance to address the former but, as just argued, the latter requires nothing more than sound judgement. This leaves open a strategy for salvaging Moore's suggestion. Perhaps the veil of ignorance thought experiment should apply not to discrete cases, as Moore suggests, but to the principles and institutions relevant to public health information; this would avoid the category error by putting the choice in the same category as Rawls's search for principles of justice.

But this strategy is disallowed in Moore's presentation because he states that, under the veil of ignorance, you know that 'privacy and public health are valuable and important for stable democratic institutions and human flourishing'. We could work at developing a version of the Rawlsian approach somewhat different to Moore's – say, under the veil of ignorance, you do not know what views you hold about democratic institutions or human flourishing – but it is hard to see the point, given that all we need for a sound judgement about children with lice or recalcitrant TB carriers are the basic facts and a moral compass.

So we are back to the familiar, well-established debate about trading-off privacy and utility in managing identifiable data. We could leave it there. But there is an intriguing research question to pursue. The debate is familiar, but are there any subtle and implicit yet pervasive and powerful influences on it? Is the debate skewed by some latent influence which should be revealed and corrected? This question is pursued here by asking whether risks and harms associated with identifiable public health information are systematically overstated; if so, this would push the pendulum of opinion towards privacy protection, at the expense of social benefit; so it must be revealed and corrected for in order to prosecute the familiar debate about identifiable public health information.

OVERSTATED HARMS

To motivate the question as to whether risks and harms associated with identifiable public health information are systematically overstated, consider a comment by Fairchild and Bayer (2016: 119): 'while the potential for misuse requires an ongoing, searching scrutiny of disease surveillance, remote or hypothetical threats should not serve to undermine this vital public health activity'. Evidently, Fairchild and Bayer are focused on surveillance, but they introduce the general question as to whether any sort of 'vital public health activity' is 'undermined by remote or hypothetical threats'.

Reductionism and Taxonomy of Harm

This would be crucial, because a debate which weighs 'threats' – informational privacy concerns about risks and harms of disclosures – against social benefit (better public health) would be skewed if the former are 'remote or hypothetical'. And this hint is made more plausible by some impressions from the relevant literature.

For one thing, lists of health informational privacy harms are strikingly small and repetitive: everyone mentions stigma and discrimination, and employment prospects and insurance (e.g. Hansson et al. 2016: 1555; Klingler et al. 2017: 295–296). This lends itself to highly reductionist accounts of informational harms. For example, in a classic statement of our theme, Hodge (2003: 663) effectively equates harms with discrimination and stigmatization:

> Protecting the privacy of individually-identifiable health data and promoting the public's health often seem at odds. Privacy advocates consistently seek to limit the acquisition, use, and disclosure of identifiable health information in governmental and private sector settings. Their concerns relate to misuses or wrongful disclosures of sensitive health data that can lead to discrimination and stigmatization against individuals.

The general impression that such accounts of health informational privacy harms are slightly glib could be put down to brevity on the part of commentators. Perhaps stigmatisation, for example, is just shorthand for all the relevant risks and harms created by identifiable health data. But consider more comprehensive taxonomies. For example, Eriksson and Helgesson's (2005) research question is about the right to withdraw one's samples from biobank research; specifically, should the right to withdraw be restricted and, if so, to what extent, and in what ways? In addressing this they clarify the 'negative effects biobank research may have' and 'the harm that may arise if sensitive personal information ends up in the wrong hands'. This ushers in a full taxonomy structured around two broad categories (p. 1072–1073). First, 'risks of harm related to biobank research' include direct and indirect physical and nonphysical harm and external and internal group harm. Second 'moral harms' (or 'wrongs') include failing to respect autonomy, privacy or integrity; violations of dignity; and treating people unjustly.

This taxonomy is questionable; for example, injustice is presented as a species of moral harm, but is illustrated by a group being 'systematically excluded from the benefits of research', which is clearly more than 'wronging' because it can have direct physical effects, so seems more like an 'external harm to groups of people'. But more to the point, the paper nicely illustrates what happens when commentators go beyond reductionist lists of health informational risks – reducing privacy harms to stigmatization, for example – to provide a fuller, more detailed analysis. Specifically, Eriksson and Helgesson use their taxonomy to explore differences between harms created by biobank versus 'human subject' research. They conclude: 'Since biobank research does not involve any risk of direct physical harm, and is likely to involve nonphysical harms of different magnitude as compared to research on living human subjects, it is reasonable to treat it as a special kind of research more akin to register research' (p. 1076).

In other words, biobank research turns out to be less risky than might initially appear and threatens fewer harms than other domains of information gathering, such as human subject research. Hence, Eriksson and Helgesson propose that withdrawal should not automatically result in anonymisation, or stopping research on identifiable samples. The details of this proposal are not so important, because the regulatory context has changed since Eriksson and Helgesson's paper; rather, the important point is that, when the risks associated with biobank research are checked against a full taxonomy of research harms, they are fewer than might be thought and fewer than other forms of information gathering.

We can go further because, as Eriksson and Helgesson's mention of 'register research' indicates, the point does not apply only to biobank research. We can extrapolate to other sorts of relevantly similar public health information. Surveillance systems, secondary uses of data, service evaluations and quality research, and so on, will turn out to be akin to biobank research in creating less risk of harm than other domains of information-gathering activities. Harms familiar from other contexts – such as direct physical harm – do not occur in the context of public health information; others, such as indirect physical harm, are less likely to occur, or, if they do, have fewer negative effects. In other words, they are, as Fairchild and Bayer suggest, 'remote or hypothetical threats'.

Health and Sensitive Information

We can take the suggestion that informational risk and privacy harms are systematically overstated in public health further, in another direction. Informational risk and sensitivity are closely related, because privacy concerns are most acute when sensitive personal data are involved; conversely, people are not so anxious about their nonsensitive personal information. And health information is often assumed to be highly sensitive. For example, GDPR 'special category data' refers to particularly sensitive personal information which requires special protections. This includes 'health data'. Processing such data is prohibited unless one of the justifications in GDPR Article 9(2) applies (ironically, given the present context, one of these is, 'processing is necessary for reasons of public interest in the area of public health' [GDPR Article 9(2)(i)]). That health data are a special category, are particularly sensitive and require special protection are reconfirmed in GDPR Article 9(4): 'Member States may maintain or introduce further conditions, including limitations, with regard to the processing of . . . data concerning health'.

Evidently, health data of the sort required for public health are seen to be highly sensitive and in need of special protection. Is this justified? Of course some health data are highly sensitive, but our research question is whether the sensitivity of identifiable public health data is systematically overstated. A banal point is that it is surely mistaken to assume that all heath information is equally sensitive. Mental health diagnoses or HIV status are very sensitive; how many teeth you have had extracted is not. To think otherwise is a form of exceptionalism; i.e. thinking that data are very sensitive just because they are health data. So we need to distinguish more from less sensitive health data and regulate accordingly, as opposed to simply assuming that all personal health information is equally and very sensitive.

Any methodology for undertaking this will prove contentious, because the sensitivity of certain sorts of health information will be contested. Nonetheless, there are a number of plausible strategies. One is to undertake elicitation studies to reveal public attitudes about the sensitivity of different sorts of health data (Stockdale, Cassell and Ford 2019). Strategies such as elicitation studies are important in sorting out which health data are genuinely sensitive, but they are refinements of the familiar privacy-utility trade-off outlined in the previous section. There is a more interesting strategy to pursue.

Sensitive Data and Conceptions of the Good

We need a handle on which health data are so sensitive that privacy protection trumps collective public health benefits. Rubel (2012) is focused on justifying public health surveillance, but the argument he presents has wider resonance. Rubel takes a broadly Rawlsian approach and, to echo the discussion in the first section of this chapter, we do not need to go deeply into Rawls's theory of justice for our present purposes. The important line of thought is as follows (Rubel 2012: 10–16).

Rubel wants a principled way of deciding whether to uphold a health information privacy claim. He distinguishes three sorts of interests. Basic interests are Rawlsian primary goods, which include 'basic rights, liberties, and opportunities, and social bases for self-respect [and] certain "natural goods," among them health' (p. 11); everyone would want more of these. Personal interests express personal preferences; for example, 'athletic recreation . . . intensive religious experiences . . . intellectual or artistic projects' (p. 11); these are idiosyncratic and often conflict. In between these, as it were, are deep personal interests, 'interests that are more weighty than (mere) personal interests but not sufficiently weighty to be considered basic' (p. 13); typically, this includes health privacy.

Rubel uses this hierarchy of interests to adjudicate health information privacy claims, i.e. to decide whether to allow or override someone's refusal to supply health information on privacy grounds. Broadly, if a privacy claim threatens a basic interest, it should be disallowed; otherwise, it can be upheld. Rubel adds subtly and nuance to this schema, and there is much to unpack and critique in this stimulating piece (we return to it in the next section, because Rubel's approach can be read as a version of Mill's harm principle). But the intriguing thing for present purposes is how Rubel argues that health privacy claims are deep personal interests (as opposed to basic or merely personal interests): 'One reason is that health information privacy is important to many persons' conception of the good' (p. 13).

The capacity to devise and pursue a 'conception of the good' is another well-known Rawlsian notion that we do not need to go into deeply here. The basic idea is that one is capable of choosing one's 'course of life' in light of an assessment of what is valuable or worthwhile, including a realistic assessment of one's options, and a 'view of our relation to the world – religious, philosophical or moral' (Rawls, 1987, p. 16). So, Rubel's suggestion is that health privacy interests are not basic interests – i.e. interests everyone has irrespective of his or her conception of the good – but they are 'deeper' than mere personal interests (individual preferences), in part because of their importance in conceptions of the good.

If this is right, it would have a notable impact on the health privacy versus utility debate by prioritising the former over the latter. A liberal society is committed to fostering the capacity of its citizens to devise and pursue a conception of the good. So if there are 'persons whose conception of the good includes (or relies on) health information privacy' (Rubel 2012: 14), there is a strong *prima facie* case for protecting it. Conversely, it will take much more by way of social utility to override health privacy claims. So, we need to interrogate this putative role of health information privacy in one's conception of the good.

Health Privacy and Conceptions of the Good

It is argued here that health information privacy can be implicated in a conception of the good – and when it is, privacy claims are very strong – but this is very unusual; for the most part, health information privacy is not part of anyone's conception of the good, so Rubel's suggestion is a case in point of overstated health informational risks and harms.

First, Rubel's discussion itself indicates that it is an exaggeration to put health information privacy in terms of a conception of the good. Having introduced the idea, Rubel goes on to say that 'the desire for health information privacy is strong, widespread, and resilient . . . there is no reason to think such a desire is based on a misplaced fear or a mistake about facts', and he lists concerns about autonomy, dignity, ill treatment, discrimination and care avoidance (p. 13–14). This is no doubt true, but it does not get us to a conception of the good. As Rubel explicitly says of care avoidance, it is important to people '*regardless* of their particular conceptions of the good [emphasis added]', and this can be extended to the other listed concerns: they are adverse consequences of health information disclosures, not integral to devising and pursuing a conception of the good. And since it is a fairly typical list, we can infer that this is the case for informational risks and harms generally; i.e. though they might be very important, they are not important because of anything as portentous as conceptions of the good.

Rubel does mention a more plausible case: 'Some people may wish not to have their identities shaped by information about their health and so may want to control who views them in terms of their health conditions and who views them without such information' (p. 14). Arguably, this does implicate a conception of the good. Identity is of a quite different order to a negative effect, such as care avoidance, because it is integral to one's capacity to devise and pursue a 'course of life'. Disclosure of such facts as that one is an HIV+ man-who-has-sex-with-men, or has a history of serious mental illness, or was not born a woman but has undergone reassignment surgery, might well 'shape identity' in ways which make it impossible to chart one's chosen course through life. In turn, it will be vital to control that information. Privacy claims in such contexts are not only very strong, they are distinctive in implicating one's conception of the good. Rubel's comment that, *ceteris paribus*, 'it would be difficult to justify the collection [of health information] as fair to the persons whose conception of the good includes (or relies on) health information privacy' (p. 14) seems entirely apposite in such cases.

Nonetheless, such cases are unusual, and most public health information is not such that disclosure shapes identity in a way that implicates conceptions of the good. Vast swathes of public health information are quotidian. As we have seen – for example, in the discussion of Eriksson and Helgesson's (2005) taxonomy – identifiable public health data create no or fewer risks and harms than is often thought, and fewer than other forms of information. Where data are such that disclosure would be damaging, the harms are straightforwardly negative effects (such as those Rubel lists). So the health informational privacy concerns and risks have been systematically overstated in a distinctive way. Rubel claims that 'health information privacy is important to many persons' conception of the good' and people's 'conception of the good includes (or relies on) health information privacy' suggest that public health information is highly sensitive. But this is only true of certain identity-shaping sorts of information. In sum, implicating conceptions of the good exaggerates the sensitivity of health data which, in turn, overstates health information risks and harms, thereby prioritising privacy protection over social benefit.

Explaining Overstated Harms

The suspicion that public health informational risks are systematically overstated would be deepened by a plausible explanation of this phenomenon. Rivera (2014) proposes one. In addressing our problematic, i.e. the 'tension between individual liberties – expressed through an emphasis on privacy protection – and collective benefit' (p. 63), Rivera focuses on secondary uses of existing data, such as electronic medical records. The drift of her argument is that progress on collective benefit should trump privacy concerns, but the part of her presentation relevant here concerns research exceptionalism which, as fully discussed in chapter 1, is a matter of treating research as more risky than relevantly similar activities, due to historical research abuses. Rivera appeals to research exceptionalism in addressing the privacy-utility trade-off:

> With regard to privacy, research exceptionalism takes the form of restrictions or prohibitions against research use of any data or materials that could potentially stigmatize the subjects. But the risk of stigma is too blunt an instrument by which to measure the likelihood or magnitude of the potential for harm. Since attitudes about privacy outside of research are evolving, in the sense that the boundaries between what is public and what is private are becoming more fluid, research regulation around the use of data should evolve, too.

Rivera's comment that, 'risk of stigma is too blunt an instrument' perfectly captures the tendency to reduce informational risks to discrimination and stigmatization, as already discussed. But the important point here is Rivera's explanation for systematically overstating public health informational risks. Historical research abuses led to research exceptionalism, which leads to exceptionalism about information acquired in research, which leads to disproportionate privacy concerns about informational risks, which leads to overstated risks of harms created by public health information. So, the suspicion that public health informational risks are overstated is supported by Rivera's explaining this phenomenon as a vestige of research exceptionalism. Hence, her conclusion is very much in keeping with the argument of this book:

> Treating research differently is harmful to public health because it slows progress on solving important problems. In this regard, our focus on privacy protection has become a hindrance to scientific progress, which cannot be justified on ethical grounds. We fuss about it disproportionately (p. 55).

APPEAL TO THE HARM PRINCIPLE

There is a different, but related, harms-based way of addressing concerns about the identifiable data required for public health. This appeals to Mill's harm principle. Since it is so familiar – not least in public health ethics – the principle can be succinctly summarised.

The harm principle concerns the legitimacy of the state's liberty-limiting interference in the lives of its citizens, and was presented by Mill (1989) in his essay *On Liberty* in 1859. The principle is often reduced – misleadingly, a point to which we return in a moment – to Mill's claim that 'the only purpose for which power can be rightfully exercised over any member of a civilized community, against his will, is to prevent harm to others' (p. 13). In other words, the only legitimation for state actions which interfere with an individual's liberty is to prevent them from harming others, i.e. from perpetrating third-party harms. In particular, and as Mill goes on to say, 'the individual's own good, either physical or moral, is not a sufficient warrant'. This rules out paternalism as a justification for liberty-limiting state interference; i.e. the state is not justified in restricting an individual's liberty on the grounds that it knows what is in that individual's best interests.

Interpreting and Applying the Harm Principle

The harm principle is influential and contentious in equal measure. On the one hand, it remains at the core of liberal political thought; and the very broad contention that harms-to-others is significant continues to inform limitations on a liberal state's authority. On the other hand, it is highly controversial. There is no consensus on how best to interpret the principle; is it a necessary and/or sufficient condition for legitimate state coercion? How expansively should the principle be interpreted (to include not only actual harms, but also risks of harms, and even some benefit)? The relative strength of the principle – including how it relates to other powerful considerations (maximising utility, minimising inequalities, proportionality and so on) – is contestable. Some commentators of a broadly liberal hue revise the framework the principle provides. For example, in developing their 'revised liberal framework [namely] the stewardship model', the Nuffield Council on Bioethics (2007: 17) was keen to point out some of Mill's 'overlooked observations'; notably, that Mill (1989: 13) endorsed state action for 'joint work necessary to the interest of society', i.e. public goods (Lee 2014: 47–49). Others object to the entire liberal context: the principle allows too much state action for libertarians, too little for communitarians (Harcourt 1999; Gostin and Gostin 2009).

The harm principle is being used here in full recognition of all these issues, but since the aim is not (yet another) treatise on the harm principle, a light touch is taken. That an action threatens harm to others provides a *prima facie* justification for restricting the agent. This core of the principle can be retained – notwithstanding that to go any further is highly contentious – and its impact can be easily illustrated by reference to public health, because a defining characteristic of public health is that it is state-backed. This immediately raises the question as to how far to allow the state to interfere in the lives of its citizens for the sake of public health goals. Mill's harm principle is obviously applicable (Holland 2015: 51-54). For example, restricting a carrier's liberty by quarantine in order to protect others from his or her disease complies with the harm principle; coercing individuals to change their dietary habits because they themselves would be better off contravenes it. Likewise, banning smoking in public places respects the harm principle because the policy is designed to protect third parties – bar staff, other customers and so on – from the effects of passive smoking. But banning smoking altogether in order to force smokers to give up because that is what is in their best interest would be paternalistic and contravene the harm principle.

These are applications of the harm principle to public health interventions, but, in the present context, the interesting – and notably under-researched – question is whether and how the harm principle applies, not to public health programmes, but to public health information. The direct application in the literature of the harm principle to the collection and use of data for public health purposes is somewhat patchy. The harm principle seems clearly relevant to some discussions, but is not applied. For example, Lee, Heilig and White (2012: 40) list harms to third parties and mention the harm principle, but do not systematically pursue this; and Angst's (2009: 172–173) discussion of whether a 'National health information exchange' should be voluntary or mandated would clearly have been enhanced by reference to the principle. On the other hand, there are some direct appeals to the principle which are misleading (Debatin 2011: 52; Al-Saggaf and Islam 2015: 289); others are incautious:

> No other moral principle that John Stuart Mill's Harm Principle is needed to justify limitations of the freedom of persons who cause, threaten to cause, or are likely to cause, information based harms to people. And Mill's Harm Principle is widely acknowledged as an uncontroversial justification for interference with individual liberty (van den Hoven 1997: 35).

More Compelling Applications of the Harm Principle

A more compelling example of an appeal to the harm principle is by the Nuffield Council on Bioethics (2007: 63–67). As part of their infection disease case study, the Council discussed surveillance which, as clarified in the taxonomy in chapter 1, is a key means of acquiring public health information. Focusing on surveillance 'to detect cases of disease that require intervention' – i.e. notifiable diseases (pp. 65–66) – the Council recognised that 'it is not required that the individual agrees to [reporting their notifiable disease] and the data passed on necessarily include information that identifies the individual', adding that some 'might take the view that consent and privacy considerations make this unacceptable'. But the council then went on to say that the 'aim of such measures is generally to prevent harm to others from the spread of disease, which means that they can be justified under the classical harm principle'. Childress (2013: 111) also explicitly applies the harm principle to public health information:

> The strongest argument for collecting information about and reporting diseases, through named reporting, is to protect others who might be at risk from individuals' uncontrolled diseases . . . These arguments represent versions of John Stuart Mill's 'harm-to-others' principle.

Both these applications of the harm principle focus on the specific case of mandatory reporting of identifiable surveillance data pertaining to notifiable communicable diseases. This is where the harm principle most neatly applies, because there is a clear third-party harm (catching the disease) and a clear rationale for the identifiable data (to facilitate case control). So, there are Millian grounds for mandating the collection of this specific sort of identifiable public health information, even if individuals would object.

We can go further, because the same Millian justification for identifiable data collection applies to any public health information which is in relevant respects like notifiable disease reporting. This might include, for example, data collection during outbreaks or emergencies. Unlike surveillance systems, these are not established or routine forms of information gathering; rather, data needs to be collected quickly and often in contravention of standard ethical and other governance constraints. In particular, mechanisms for ensuring anonymity might not be in place – due to the need to collect information quickly – or not desirable given the goals of monitoring and containing the event. The collection of data would be justified on the same grounds as in the case of mandatory reporting of notifiable diseases: there is a clear threat of harm to others from the failure to manage the emergency or contain the outbreak, and a clear rationale for the rapid collection of identifiable data. The same line of thought would apply to any isomorphic public health information.

Further Applications

Can we go even further? For example, might the harm principle be the basis for an argument in favour of using identifiable novel forms of information, such as social media data, for public health purposes (McDonald et al. 2016)? The main objection to doing so – i.e. to applying the harm principle to public health information beyond the specific case of communicable disease notification – is a *reductio ad absurdum* argument. If we justify lots of public health information by the harm principle, we allow lots of liberty-limiting state interference for public health goals, in the form of illiberal public health programmes, such as banning smoking. But there is a significant difference between public health programmes and public health information. Coercive public health programmes are troubling because they are the imposition by the state of behaviours and lifestyle choices on supposedly free individuals; by contrast, coercive public health data collection leaves intact the individual's freedom to live life how he or she pleases. Bluntly, there is a significant difference between the state's telling someone whether he or she can smoke versus the state telling that person to tell the state whether he or she smokes. The former is up to the individual, whereas the latter is merely information about his or her freely made decision. So the *reductio* objection to applying the harm principle to public health information beyond communicable disease notification founders.

Given this, the question persists: to what extent can the acquisition and use of identifiable data for public health purposes be justified by the harm principle, beyond communicable disease notification and relevantly similar cases? The way Rubel (2012) frames this question is very useful. As discussed in the previous section, Rubel develops 'conditions under which individuals may justifiably exercise individual privacy claims that conflict with public health goals', taking a 'basic interests approach' which he develops into what he calls the 'unreasonable exercise' argument. The latter turns on the effects on others of an individual exercising his or her privacy claim, and culminates with:

> In cases in which a person's exercising a claim to privacy in health information with respect to state agencies is likely to cause others serious injury, illness, or death, it is justified to restrict that claim. This is the basic condition of the permissibility of mandatory collection of personal information (pp. 16–17).

Rubel's argument does not mention Mill's harm principle, but Childress (2013: 111) is right to call it 'a version of the Millian principle' because the 'unreasonable exercise' argument can be put in terms of third-party harms, as follows. Identifiable information is required by public health. Individuals have legitimate claims to privacy in health information. We need a principled way of adjudicating between these. Rubel's approach is a version of the harm principle: whether an individual's health privacy claim should be upheld turns on whether it threatens to seriously harm others by threatening their basic interests, i.e. 'is likely to cause others serious injury, illness, or death'. This provides a template for adjudicating between public health and informational privacy. For example, Rubel juxtaposes TB and diabetes, arguing that it is easier to justify mandatory surveillance of the former than the latter, because it is a communicable disease, so notification is more likely to avoid serious third-party harms ('serious injury, illness, or death').

To reiterate, this is a template, not an algorithm. How the harm principle applies in specific cases will depend on numerous factors, such as how to interpret the principle. To illustrate, Childress (2013: 111) comments, 'narrowly understood [the harm principle] offers no warrant for the diabetes surveillance and intervention program, since diabetes is not communicable' (which echoes Rubel's juxtaposition, just mentioned). But Childress immediately goes on to say that 'there may be other harms to others in a much more interdependent society than existed in Mill's day . . . the financial burdens associated with diseases are borne in part by taxpayers'. This dialectic is familiar from the previous discussion about how widely to interpret the harm principle. 'Narrowly understood', as Childress puts it, the harm principle requires something like 'clear and present danger', such as passing on a communicable disease; interpreted more widely, the harm principle would justify a greater range of liberty-limiting interventions on grounds such as the third-party harm of increased burden on taxpayers. So, for example, illiberal policies such as an outright ban on smoking or mandatory regular exercise would be justified, because smoking and a sedentary lifestyle create health needs that can only be met by higher taxes, which is a form on third-party harm. Applied to public health information, lots of infringement of informational privacy would be justified by reference to third-party harms if these – and the principle based on them – are more broadly construed.

A sensible position is to leave this moot. As mentioned a number of times, applications of the harm principle to public health information – as opposed to interventions or programmes – is an under-researched area, so this can be read as an invitation for further reflection. The important points are these. The harm principle can be – indeed, has been – applied to specific forms of identifiable public health information, namely, notifiable disease reporting. This can be extended to other forms of identifiable public health information which are relevantly similar to notifiable disease reporting; for example, identifiable data collection during emergencies and outbreaks. How much further the harm principle can be used to disallow privacy claims and collect identifiable public health data is moot, as it depends on how the principle is interpreted, the sorts and severity of third-party harms and the weight of the principle relative to other considerations. In sum, the harm principle is a promising approach to the ethics and governance of public health information; it forms part of the cumulative case presented in this chapter for using identifiable data for public health purposes.

CONCLUDING REMARKS

This chapter has focused on identifiable data because these are required in public health. In keeping with the overall aim of this book, identifiable public health information has been defended from the overly restrictive effects of heightened privacy concerns. The first strategy was to reveal ways in which the risks and harms associated with identifiable data are systematically overstated in the public health literature. The assumption that identifiable public health information is very risky in lots of ways is unwarranted – for example, very little of the data required for public health is sensitive, or constituents of anyone's conception of the good – and to think otherwise is a form of health data exceptionalism. The second strategy was to make a direct appeal to the harm principle to justify the acquisition and use of identifiable public health information. The principle clearly works for paradigm cases, such as notifiable disease reporting; and it was argued that the principle can be applied further, at least to include information gathering, such as in emergencies, which is relevantly similar to disease notification, and perhaps even further.

As a final remark, it is very important to reiterate exactly what is being argued for in this chapter. Nothing in this chapter is complacent about the informational risks and privacy harms created by identifiable information. That health informational risks are systematically overstated and the harm principle is an underused way of justifying identifiable public health data are entirely compatible with there being some very high risks and serious harms created by identifiable information. The negative effects of identifiable data can be hugely detrimental to individuals' well-being, and data disclosure can ruin people's lives. Of course it is vital to identify such cases and to prioritise privacy protection over collective benefit. Nonetheless, these are fewer and more isolated cases than the literature would suggest; we should resist inferring from these that all public health information is equally risky and disallow what Fairchild and Bayer called 'remote or hypothetical threats' from undermining vital public health activity.

Chapter 6

Consent

None of the foregoing discussion denies that some public health data are highly sensitive, create significant informational risks and cause serious privacy harms. These need to be managed, so the next two chapters address the two most prominent approaches, centring on consent and trust, respectively. The argument regarding consent in this chapter is as follows.

Gaining consent to gather public health information is problematic, mainly because it would be impracticable or distort data. Distinguishing types of public health information by reference to the consent requirement helps to address this problem. This distils the hard consent problem in public health down to further research use of personal health data. The debate about further uses is dominated by competing consent models and is at an impasse, so a novel approach is recommended here. Ballantyne and Schaefer (2018) have recently argued that the consent requirement on further uses of personal health data is overridden by a duty to participate in health data research. Their argument is endorsed but is essentially negative, their main point being that objections to a general duty to participate in research do not apply to the specific case of further research on personal health data. So this already strong negative argument is strengthened in this chapter by a positive free riding argument for a duty to contribute data. In addition, Ballantyne and Schaefer focused solely on personal health data, but, arguably, the duty to participate extends to contributing other sorts of public health data. Two are discussed: biological samples used for future biobank research and novel forms of information, such as social media data.

PUBLIC HEALTH'S CONSENT PROBLEM

Voluntary informed consent is the traditional mechanism for eliciting participation in risky activities. The basic rationale is to give control over the decision to participate to the individual involved. But the consent requirement fits public health information badly. This is repeatedly raised in the literature on public health information. To illustrate by reference to the taxonomy presented in chapter 1, all standard forms of public health practice – surveillance, data collection during emergencies and service evaluation – create much discussed ethical tensions around consent (Lee 2014; Mitra and Sethi 2016; Baily et al. 2006), as do distinctive public health data sources (health activity data, biobanks and novel forms of health information: Hoffman and Podgurski 2012; Virani and Longstaff 2015; Vayena, Mastroianni and Kahn 2012), and the cross-cutting themes of secondary analysis, data linkage and 'big data' (Lowrance 2003; Lipworth et al. 2017).

The specific details of the problem with consent vary between these forms of public health data, but two general themes run throughout. First, acquiring individual voluntary informed consent is impracticable. In particular, the sheer size of data sets required for public health makes it impossible to acquire individual consent. Second, imposing a consent requirement would frustrate the public health goals for which the information was gathered. Regarding the latter, there is an ongoing dispute as to whether obtaining consent results in consent bias – i.e. information is distorted because the group that consents to provide it is relevantly different to the group that refuses (Rothstein and Shoben 2013) – but whether or not this specific type of selection bias exists, the general point that insisting on consent threatens to distort or corrupt public health data is widely accepted.

The upshot is a dilemma between the consent requirement and public health information. Given that privacy concerns are heightened in the 'information age', it would be unsurprising if the response to a data-consent dilemma were a shift away from unconsented data collection on privacy grounds. In turn – and as has long been recognised (Coleman, Evans and Barrett 2003) – this is detrimental to public health. So we need ways of addressing the data-consent dilemma that protects public health information.

CATEGORISING PUBLIC HEALTH DATA BY REFERENCE TO CONSENT

The strategy pursued here distinguishes public health information–gathering activities by reference to the consent requirement. There are four categories, which cross-cut the taxonomy of public health information presented in chapter 1.

Traditional Consent Requirement

First, some public health data collection is traditional in that it uses established study designs and recruits individual participants who can and should be allowed to consent to participate. For example, RCTs (randomised control trials) are frequently used to acquire public health data. It is natural to map this onto the first category in the taxonomy of public health information presented in chapter 1, i.e. research. But although research was characterised in chapter 1 as 'controlled trials and experimental techniques: in sum, the scientific method as applied in the field of public health', standard study designs can be used for other public health purposes, such as service evaluations and quality improvement. The most important feature of this category is that the consent requirement on these activities is not distinctive of public health, but generic, familiar and standard, so there is no consent problem for public health *per se*.

But it is worth adding that the traditional requirement of individual voluntary informed consent to participate in studies using established designs (such as RCTs) is the subject of ongoing critique. The backdrop to this is the 'triumph of the minimal conception of individual autonomy that identifies it with informed consent requirements' (O'Neill 2002: 47). Specifically, consent processes are said not to be fit for purpose, being mechanistic, neither satisfactorily voluntary nor properly informed, and they are not genuinely protective of individual autonomy. We do not need to go into this here, other than to note that the critique instigated a gradual overhaul of traditional consent requirements which takes the onus off individual voluntary informed consent and recommends more intellectually and practically convincing consent mechanisms, all of which is conducive to public health information. But the main point for present purposes is that there is no consent problem regarding this first category of public health data, over and above that which applies to all such traditional forms of information gathering.

No Consent Requirement

The second category comprises public health information–gathering activities on which there is no consent requirement. Gelinas, Wertheimer and Miller (2016) suggest a general justification for research without consent: 'socially valuable research is justified without the consent of the participants if the research stands to infringe no right of the participants and it is impracticable to obtain consent' (p. 35). That public health information is 'socially valuable' is a given, and we will return to the impracticability condition, so the important point to explicate here is about rights. According to Gelinas, Wertheimer and Miller, the 'most basic function of consent is to waive rights of control, allowing others to interact with us in ways that would otherwise be wrong' (p. 36). For example, injections require consent because sticking needles into someone threatens his or her right to bodily integrity. Given this, 'it will be relatively easy to justify research without consent when such research does not violate the rights of subjects' (p. 35). Gelinas, Wertheimer and Miller's account of the right to consent is not contentious, so it can ground and illustrate this second category of public health information, i.e. data collection that does not require consent.

Conveniently enough, the first case of research which does not require consent that Gelinas, Wertheimer and Miller discuss is a standard public health information–gathering practice, namely, 'quality improvement research' (pp 37–39). So here we have an illustration of public health data that do not require consent. But we can go further, because Gelinas, Wertheimer and Miller's justification for quality improvement research without consent seems clearly to apply to other public health information, such as routine surveillance systems. The three conditions they mention are met: that surveillance is socially valuable is a given; the impracticability of obtaining consent for routine surveillance is obvious; and given the way they operate, routine surveillance systems do not stand to infringe population members' rights. Gelinas, Wertheimer and Miller's line of thought might be taken even further in the public health context – in discussions around big data and consent, for example – but this will be left moot; the point here is that there is a secondary category of public health information, i.e. data collection which does not require consent, which includes at least quality improvement research and routine surveillance.

Overriding Consent

For the third category of public health data, Gelinas, Wertheimer and Miller (2016) are again instructive. They 'endorse a second rationale for justifiably waiving consent: research that does infringe participant rights can be justified if the gravity of the rights infringement is minor and outweighed by the expected social value of the research and if it is impracticable to obtain consent' (p. 35). They apply this rationale to research with stored samples (pp. 39–40). But as their judicious discussion illustrates, this was bound to be inconclusive: 'Whether stored samples can permissibly be used without consent cannot be resolved without a deeper normative investigation into the rights at issue'. In other words, if no rights are at issue, research with stored samples does not require consent; if robust rights are at issue, research with stored samples does require consent; so whether or not stored samples require consent depends on a prior discussion of the sort and strengths of rights violated by biobank research. Hence, we will return to the vexed issue of consent to further uses of stored biological samples.

There is a much more straightforward application of Gelinas, Wertheimer and Miller's second rationale for justifiably waiving consent: data collection during public health emergencies. This clearly fits their schema. The sorts of information-gathering activities used in emergency situations would, under normal circumstances, require ethical scrutiny and governance oversight. This is captured by Gelinas, Wertheimer and Miller's account, because such activities threaten to infringe rights – to privacy, bodily integrity and so on – which grounds a right to control expressed as a consent requirement. But waiving consent is justified. First, it is easy to see how the 'gravity of the rights infringement' might well be 'outweighed by expected social value', because public health emergencies threaten catastrophe. Second, the impracticability requirement is met, because the rapidity with which emergency and outbreak situations develop precludes the usual niceties around obtaining consent. Again, this line of thought might be taken even further than data collection during public health emergencies – by definition, all public health activities promise very high expected social value – but we can leave this moot here. The point is that there is a third category of public health data, which includes data collection during emergencies, in which the consent requirement is outweighed by social value.

Hard Cases

So far it has proved difficult to see a serious consent problem for public health *per se*. But there is a fourth category of genuinely hard cases. A simple way to introduce these is to negate the previous three categories. Unlike the first category, hard cases are distinctive to public health; unlike the second category, they do impose a consent requirement; and unlike the third category, the consent requirement is not obviously outweighed by social value. Members of this fourth category include further uses of personal data to which individuals have not consented. A case in point, encountered a moment ago (and to which we will return), is further use of biobanked samples to support public health, because this seems to require consent, and the consent requirement may well not be outweighed by the social value of a study. Likewise, personal health data, including electronic medical records, are important resources for public health; but their secondary or further use seems to impose a consent requirement not necessarily outweighed by the social value that accrues. Meeting the consent requirement on such further uses of data is impracticable (given the size of data sets) and undesirable (because it would result in data corruption), so we get to the nub of the consent problem in public health.

MODELS OF CONSENT

This dilemma has generated a sizeable literature which has reached an impasse. Specific features on the terrain of the debate are confusing, but the general topography is clear. In response to hard cases, three models or frameworks for consent to further use of personal health data are salient. First, the specific consent model requires consent to each use. Second, broad consent models allow individuals to set parameters around uses of their data; consent is not required for each use within those parameters. Third, open consent allows unrestricted use of personal data without further consent.

This tripartite reconstruction is deceptively simple. For one thing, there is a proliferation of variants on each model and some terminological confusion. For example, 'specific consent' is also called 'narrow consent', and forms of dynamic consent are, in effect, specific consent models. Tiered or categorical consent are variants on broad consent; and blanket consent is sometimes presented as a form of broad consent, sometimes as equivalent to open consent. As this last point suggests, the three models are best thought of as on a continuum – roughly, from full to some to no consent – along which some types of consent can move. For example, the broader the consent in the middle of the continuum, the more it resembles open consent. And in addition to these three innovative models, some writers advocate traditional consent mechanisms, such as opt-out versus opt-in or presumed consent.

The Trilemma

None of these details are as important as the fact that there is a trilemma between these three consent models. In other words, each model captures something important but is vulnerable to criticism. This can be quickly illustrated with some standard moves in the debate. Specific consent is attractive in allowing individuals full control, but it is impracticable. Broad consent is more practicable in allowing data to be used without individuals having to consent to each use, but is not really consent because individuals are not informed about specific uses of their data. Open consent would achieve lots of public utility but clearly fails to respect individual autonomy and the right to control. All these standard moves are queried by advocates defending one or another of these models; but the debate is unresolved, and there is no consensus on the correct consent model, because, at root, this is a trilemma.

Because this is a trilemma, it was inevitable that the debate would reach an impasse. To illustrate, it was only a matter of time before someone opposed selecting between these three equally unsatisfactory models and proposed combining them. Ploug and Holm (2015, 2015a) duly obliged by presenting 'meta consent', which amounts to asking individuals for their preferred model of consent to categories of research. Ploug and Holm's advocacy of meta consent includes a more in-depth theoretical discussion (2016) and examples of practical application (2017, 2017a; cf. Van Howe et al. 2019). But that the debate is at an impasse is demonstrated by the fact that meta consent has already elicited rejoinders by writers sympathetic to first order consent models.

For example, Budin-Ljøsne et al. (2015) are advocates of dynamic consent, so their 'rapid response' to Ploug and Holm (2015a) critiqued meta consent from that perspective. Even more recently, Manson (2018, 2019) – who has defended broad consent from a 'right to control' problem – criticised meta consent for being impractical and pointed out that there is no grounding for an obligation to provide meta consent. The details of these responses – or Ploug and Holm's replies – are not material. The important point is that this is a predictable dialectic: from trilemma to impasse to meta consent to a return to impasse. There is no real prospect of resolving this trilemma by achieving convergence on any one of the items on the menu of consent models, so we need a novel approach.

A DUTY TO CONTRIBUTE DATA

The approach pursued here is that the consent requirement is overridden by a duty or obligation to allow further uses of personal data. The background to this is a long-standing dispute over the duty or obligation to participate in biomedical research. To quickly sketch this background, Jonas (1976) was an early sceptic – largely because he did not think of medical progress itself as morally required – Caplan (1984) was an early advocate. The subsequent debate was stimulated by seminal arguments for a duty to participate in medical research presented separately by Rhodes (2005) and Harris (2005). Each of these elicited criticisms and sustained responses. For example, Brassington (2007, 2014) and Shapshay and Pimple (2007) take on Harris, who duly responded (Chan and Harris 2009). Likewise, objections to Rhodes's argument – for example, Allhoff (2005) – elicited reiterations of her view (Rhodes 2005[a], 2017). Advocates of a duty to participate in biomedical research have presented other arguments (Schaefer, Emanuel and Wertheimer 2009); by contrast, detractors suggest alternative ways of acquiring participation (Mehlman, Kodish and Berg 2018).

From Biomedical Research to Public Health Information

There is no intention to engage directly with this debate about a duty to participate in biomedical research. Rather, the point for present purposes is that there are perennial hints in this literature of a corresponding duty to contribute to public health information gathering. This could be discerned at the start of the controversy. For example, in his philosophical comment on human experimentation, Jonas (1976) queries the view that society can ill afford not to pursue medical experimentation on human subjects (pp. 226–231). He points out that society – though not, of course, individual patients – would survive and flourish perfectly well without the benefits of medical experimentation: 'If cancer, heart disease, and other organic, noncontagious ills…continue to exact their toll at the normal rate of incidence…society can go on flourishing in every way' (p. 228). But he immediately goes on explore what 'by contrast…society cannot afford', citing 'epidemic rage…debilitating state of general health…endemic malaria…and averting disaster [which] extend into long-term prevention' (pp. 228–229). These are central public health issues. So Jonas was sceptical about medical experimentation on human subjects, because he recognised that society can afford not to pursue advancement in clinical medicine; but his scepticism did not extend to preventive public health and the information gathering it requires.

This segue from biomedical research to public health is evident in more recent literature. For example, Rhodes's (2005) original argument mentioned 'population studies…crucial for identifying the genetic component of disease and for improving the efficacy of medical therapy' (2005: 15). Likewise, in replies to comments on that paper, Rhodes (2005[a]: W17) explicitly mentions that 'the kind of population-based interventions that public health measures address requires information from populations', and goes on: 'Preventive medicine, disease control, public health, emergency triage, and mass casualty medicine all include a focus on the interests of populations'. Again these are central public health issues.

Segueing from biomedical research to public health information is even more apparent in a recent iteration of Rhodes's (2017) view:

> Registries for evaluating the long-term effectiveness of an intervention as well as the complications from receiving it, and population studies that aim at following health trends (e.g., changes in the microbiome within a community) or

> the geographic distribution of disease (e.g., public health surveillance of the Zika virus), or determining the impact of various environmental factors on an entire population, all require the participation of everyone in the relevant group. That is because missing data can distort the result and lead to the adoption of inappropriate responses (p. 321).

And in their engagement with the ongoing dispute between Harris and Brassington (cited previously), Forsberg, Hansson and Eriksson (2014) refer to 'stored tissue samples and data in medical records and registries', commenting that, 'when participation is not universal, registries and biobanks are affected by both those who participate and those who do not, resulting in incomplete information and data-bank bias' (pp. 325–326).

An Argument for a Duty to Contribute Public Health Data

So, whether or not there is a duty to participate in biomedical research, the literature on that controversy hints at a cognate argument for a duty to contribute to public health information gathering. Ballantyne and Schaefer (2018) make this explicit by arguing for an ethical duty to participate in health data research. Specifically, Ballantyne and Schaefer focus on the use of personal health data from clinical records for secondary research. They argue as follows.

The general duty to participate in research is controversial. But three of the most powerful objections to such a general duty do not apply in the specific case of secondary uses of health data. So even if there is no general duty, there could be a specific obligation to contribute one's health data for secondary research purposes. Using identifiable health data for secondary research imposes a consent requirement. Currently, this can be waived only if it is demonstrated that obtaining consent would be impractical. But given their argument for a duty to contribute, Ballantyne and Schaefer conclude that the consent requirement for using personal health data for secondary research purposes can be waived even if it would be practicable to obtain consent.

Evidently, the core of Ballantyne and Schaefer's argument is that three strong objections to a general duty to participate in research do not hold against the specific duty to contribute health data for secondary purposes. Here there is a dialectical oddity. The first objection to a general duty to participate in medical research they discuss is that the benefits which accrue are unequally distributed. Ballantyne and Schaefer rightly point out that this objection does not apply to heath data research, because everyone stands to benefit, and proportionately so, from resultant public health gains. The second objection to a general duty they discuss is that medical research is invasive, so it threatens direct violation of bodily integrity. Again, as Ballantyne and Schaefer rightly point out, this does not apply to secondary uses of health data. But the putative third objection is that 'enforcing the obligation to contribute health data for research could significantly undermine public trust in researchers as well as health systems' (p. 394). And this is not an objection to a general duty to participate, but to their own proposal; in fact, one they think 'is the most significant barrier to our proposal'. Although this is dialectically odd, it is not a deep problem. In response to this barrier, Ballantyne and Schaefer's proposed 'regulatory model aims to minimise harm and promote transparency and public trust', including requisite regulatory changes and an enhanced public good test. These are perfectly feasible, so this dialectical oddity is not a substantive difficulty for their view.

Support for the Argument

A practical point strongly supports the argument for a duty to contribute public health data. The obvious practical problems in enforcing a duty to participate in medical research were recognised early in the debate (Allhoff 2005); exactly who is going to be forced into a clinical trial, and when and how? What system of conscripted participation stands any chance of being implemented? Consequently: 'Even among proponents of the duty to participate, few support conscription of competent adults into interventional research' (Ballantyne and Schaefer 2018: 392). There are no such 'conscription' problems in the case of health data for further uses. Most standard forms of gathering such public health information – for example, electronic medical records, surveillance data, health activity data and so on – are routine and ongoing and do not require anything like a system of conscription.

Elicitation studies also support the argument. For example, Hepgul et al. (2019) elicited patient and public attitudes towards using personal health information for research. Their informants did mention caveats – that data is properly de-identified and there are 'adequate information governance arrangements and effective information technology safeguards', and so on – but these were addressed by Ballantyne and Schaefer. Hence, Hepgul et al. find it 'reassuring that the perspectives and considerations raised by Ballantyne and Schaefer and the wider research community are on the whole reflective of those raised by patients and the public in our consultation'.

In passing, it is worth pointing out that, despite their evidence in support of Ballantyne and Schaefer's argument, Hepgul et al. still press for 'the provision of opt-out processes where possible'. This seems to be motivated by concerns about violations of autonomy, but the point of establishing a duty to contribute personal health data is that this overrides autonomy-based refusal;

furthermore, to allow opt-outs would reintroduce the two main features which drove the consent problem in the first place, namely, impracticability and data distortion. Likewise, Hepgul et al. comment: 'Framing the use of health data in research as an obligation neglects the reality that some patients view the use of their data as positive and have a desire to give back'; but it is crucial that this is an obligation because, otherwise, we are back to individual preferences which cannot practicably be taken into account and, if they were, would distort data.

Ballantyne and Schaefer's view has practical and empirical support, and since it so clearly concords with the approach taken in this book, it is fully endorsed here. But it needs to be augmented. Ballantyne and Schaefer's argument is primarily negative, because their main premise is that objections to a general duty to participate in research do not apply to the specific case of further uses of personal health data. They do canvass three grounds for a general duty to participate in research – namely, beneficence, fairness and civic responsibility to support public goods – but they remain 'neutral' on these. Also, their discussion is clearly premised on the assumption that research is of great social benefit; but to assume that the value of research is greater than our 'interests in controlling access to and use of personal health information' would beg the question. So, given its dialectal structure, Ballantyne and Schaefer's argument is open to the rejoinder that, even if they are right that objections to a general duty do not hold against the specific duty to contribute personal health data, still there might not be this specific duty. Evidently, what is required is a positive reason for taking Ballantyne and Schaefer's view.

A FREE RIDING ARGUMENT FOR A DUTY TO CONTRIBUTE PUBLIC HEALTH DATA

The suggestion here is that there is a strong free riding argument (FRA) for a specific duty to contribute personal health data. The basic idea in any FRA is straightforward: free riders enjoy a benefit without contributing to its creation. This is morally objectionable, so there is a duty to contribute to creating the benefit. In turn, it is justifiable to coerce contribution without consent. The standard example is literal free riding: not paying a fare for a bus ride is to free ride on the contributions of others; this is morally objectionable, so there is a duty to pay one's fare. Hence it is justifiable to coerce payment without consent. Applied in the present context, not contributing personal health data for further use is to enjoy the benefits from further uses of people's health data. This is morally objectionable, so there is a duty to contribute health data. Hence, it is justifiable to undertake further research on health data without consent. The closest Ballantyne and Schaefer get to this is their appeal to fairness as one of the three grounds for a general duty to participate in research they canvass; so, the FRA argument presented here can be read as a non-neutral development of this grounding.

Empirical Support for the FRA

The FRA for a duty to contribute personal data for public health purposes will be defended here in two ways: one empirical, the other theoretical. Empirical support is provided by Slegers et al.'s (2015) study of willingness to participate in epidemiological research. This was a mixed-methods qualitative study comprised of focus groups and semistructured interviews with stakeholders, including members of the public. The interesting finding for present purposes is:

> Consistent with the 'free rider' ethical argument . . . interviewees described a sense of obligation about making their routinely collected data available to research if they had used government health services. For example, Mike from focus group D with the general public remarked:
>
>> You could say the correct ethical position surely should be that if you have a medical condition then you accept as part of the cost of your treatment that you would be happy to provide the results or be put on a registry for the purposes of advancing medical knowledge and you consent, it ought to be part of the bargain in the knowledge that the information won't be made available to door-to-door salesmen or marketing.
>
> An epidemiologist from a government health department expressed this argument as a reason why consent should not always be sought:
>
>> where people have used government services, maybe they have an obligation to society, they may not recognise it, but their data should be available for understanding the impact of various factors on health . . . (Paul, epidemiologist).

Theoretical Support: The Kantian Version of the Argument

In addition to empirical support, the FRA for a duty to contribute personal health data for further uses is theoretically robust. Here it is important to distinguish two forms of the FRA, labelled here the fairness and Kantian forms. The difference between the two lies in what makes free riding morally objectionable.

As the label suggests, the fairness version locates the wrongness of free riding in unfairness. This appeals to the fairness principle (Hart 1955; Rawls 1971) and is expressed in various ways: to enjoy benefits without contributing is unfair to those who create the good, or offends a principle of justice; sometimes it is captured in terms of social cooperation, social contract or the production of public goods, which establish a duty on each beneficiary to contribute their fair share (Scanlon 1998). By contrast, the Kantian version of FRAs characterises the wrongness of free riding in terms of (unsurprisingly) Kant's ethics. Kant's first formulation of the categorical imperative requires rational moral agents to act according to maxims they can will to be universal laws. The free rider's maxim, enjoy a benefit without contributing to its creation, fails the universalisability test.

Incidentally, this failure can be put in terms of either a contradiction in conception or a contradiction in the will, depending on how these are interpreted. In terms of a contradiction in the will, the free rider wills both the universalisation of the maxim, enjoy a benefit without contributing to its creation (so they can enjoy the benefit), and that the maxim does not hold universally (so they can make an exception of themselves), which is contradictory. But on some interpretations, free riders create a contradiction in conception. For example, on Korsgaard's (1996: 92–93) 'practical contradiction interpretation', free riding creates a contradiction in conception because the agent would be unable to act on their maxim in a world in which it is universalised (there would be no benefit for them to enjoy). In Kantian terms, which sort of contradiction free riding creates in turn determines whether there is an imperfect or perfect duty to others to contribute, but we do not need to decide this here.

So, there are two forms of the FRA – the fairness and Kantian – which lead to two versions of the FRA for a duty to contribute personal data. The free rider enjoys the benefits of further uses of data without contributing his or her own. In the fairness version, what makes this morally objectionable is that it is unfair; in the Kantian version, what makes this morally objectionable is that the agent has contradicted himself or herself by acting on a non-universalisable maxim. The original controversy over a duty to participate in biomedical research, reported previously, was pursued almost entirely in terms of fairness. For example, Rhodes (2005), Harris (2005) and their interlocutors hardly refer to Kant, and where they do, either the universalisability test is not mentioned (an exception is Allhoff [2005], who explicitly cites Kant's view that 'we may only act on universalizable maxims [which] prohibits free-riding') or quickly drops out of the discussion (van den Hoven 2012: 155). But the focus here is on the Kantian version because, arguably, the Kantian FRA for a duty to contribute personal data is stronger than the fairness version. After all, whilst duty can be grounded in fairness, this only results in *prima facie* duties which can be overridden by other considerations. By contrast, the Kantian FRA establishes a categorical imperative, i.e. a binding duty.

Theoretical support for this Kantian FRA for a duty to contribute personal health data is gained by referring to a more established FRA in public health ethics, namely, the FRA for a duty to participate in vaccine programmes. Menzel (1995) presented a Kantian FRA for a duty to participate in vaccination programmes, which was further discussed by Holland (2015: 201–210) and Schröder-Bäck and Martakis (2015). This FRA for vaccine compliance has the now-familiar structure: vaccine refusers enjoy the benefits of herd immunity created by others. This is morally objectionable, so there is a duty to get vaccinated. Hence, mandatory or coercive vaccination policies are justifiable. The important point is how this vaccination FRA fails. Put as a Kantian FRA, the argument turns on whether the agent's maxim is universalisable. But what is their maxim? Obviously, if their maxim is, enjoy a benefit without contributing to its creation, this fails the universalisability test, and we have an FRA for a duty to get vaccinated. But, as is well documented, there are a number of well-known and much discussed principled reasons for declining vaccines, including a concern to protect one's children and religious and philosophical objections (May and Silverman 2005; Bernheim et al. 2013: 152ff). In other words, the vaccine refuser might be acting on various maxims, some of which will pass the universalisability test.

As mentioned, this objection to the FRA for coercive vaccination policies is well documented. Menzel (1995: 114–115) was getting at this by asking after 'the proper reference of universalisation'. Holland (2015: 205–206) makes the same point and suggests that, whatever the proper referent is, it must be a maxim and not (as Menzel seemed to suggest) an action. The significance of this objection to the FRA for coercive vaccination is perfectly captured by the Nuffield Council on Bioethics (2007: 56):

> It could be suggested that individuals who are not vaccinated are free-riders. . . . However, we find this suggestion unhelpful for understanding the complexities raised by vaccines. Although it is true that people pursuing such self-serving strategies would receive a personal benefit, not all who object to vaccinations or refuse them are motivated in this way. There are a range of other reasons for their objections: for example, people may not be convinced of the need for the vaccine, or may be concerned about its effects on themselves or their children.

The point for present purposes is that this is a strong objection to an FRA for compulsory vaccination, but it simply does not apply to an FRA for a duty to contribute one's personal data for public health purposes. The reason is that there are not numerous principled reasons for withholding personal data from further uses; rather, there is just one plausible maxim, namely, protect one's informational privacy whilst enjoying the benefits of others' contributions. This is clearly a non-universalisable maxim, so fails the universalisability test. There do not seem to be any alternative maxims, equivalent to the concern to protect one's children or religious or philosophical objections, which govern some vaccine noncompliance. In Kantian terms, the noncontributor is making an exception of himself or herself. After all, everyone has privacy concerns; by enjoying the relevant public health benefits, the withholder is free riding on the willingness of others to run privacy risks.

OBJECTIONS

Having provided empirical and theoretical support, there is space to consider two objections to the FRA for a duty to contribute public health data for further use without consent. The first objection appeals to the distinction between voluntary and nonvoluntary benefits. The agent who withholds personal data could argue that he or she is not a free rider because he or she never wanted the benefits that accrue from others' data contributions (i.e. these are nonvoluntary benefits). This raises the issue as to whether a noncontributor who has benefits foisted on him or her is free riding, the literature on which is copious and unresolved (Cullity [1995: 9], for example, endorses 'an *extended* Principle of Fairness – one according to which it can be unfair to refuse to contribute to the production of benefits that have been conferred upon one nonvoluntarily').

But we can simply circumvent the issue. For one thing, whatever the outcome of the voluntary versus nonvoluntary benefits debate, it is surely plausible that most people do want public health benefits. Public health is about protecting and promoting health; this is something most people clearly want. So, probably, the noncontributor does want to enjoy public health benefits. And if this is unconvincing, we can appeal to the fact that public health benefits are shared. Even if we are dealing with a genuinely recalcitrant noncontributor, i.e. someone who really does not want the benefits for himself or herself, he or she probably wants them for his or her children, or loved ones generally. So, given that the noncontributor probably does voluntarily enjoy the benefits, the objection which trades on the distinction between voluntary and nonvoluntary benefits founders.

The second objection is that the argument proves too much, because endorsing an FRA for a duty to contribute health data for secondary use entails a general duty to participate in research, including biomedical research. But here we can repeat the move Ballantyne and Schaefer made and point out relevant dissimilarities between further uses of health data and biomedical research. The two Ballantyne and Schaefer discussed are clearly apposite: biomedical research creates unequally distributed benefits and threatens bodily integrity. And to these can be added a whole host of other features of biomedical research cited in the debate about a duty to participate, which are not shared with public health. For example, medical research participants are often paid for their participation (Allhoff 2005); the recipient of benefits of research does contribute to their creation, not by participation, but in other ways, such as paying taxes which fund research (Brassington 2007); and there is usually a time lag between medical research and its benefits, so contributors and beneficiaries are nonidentical (Shapshay and Pimple 2007). Such features make nonparticipation in medical research disanalogous to classic free riding, which undermines an FRA for a duty to participate. After all, the less nonparticipation in medical research resembles classic free riding, the harder it is to base a duty to contribute on an FRA. So the FRA for a duty to contribute health data for secondary use does not entail an FRA for a duty to participate in biomedical research, and the objection that the argument proves too much founders.

There is a third objection which, though not fatal, does require a caveat on the FRA for a duty to contribute personal health data. A standard argument for a consent requirement on further uses of personal data is that information might be used in ways to which the individual has principled – political, ethical, religious, philosophical – objections. Examples familiar from the literature include antiabortionists objecting to their data being used to facilitate terminations and lots of people objecting to their data being used for commercial purposes. To put this standard argument in the Kantian terms of the discussion in this chapter, these principled objections are maxims which the agent could will to be universal laws, so the Kantian form of the FRA for a duty to contribute health data fails. Another way of putting it is that the standard argument about principled objections to contributing data makes the FRA about personal health information parallel to the FRA about vaccine compliance; in both cases, the FRA fails because the noncompliant agent is objecting on principle as opposed to free riding.

This is a significant point, but there are two things to say in response. First, it is important to bear the present context in mind. The FRA is for a duty to contribute personal health data for basic public health purposes, i.e. protecting and promoting the population's health, and reducing health inequalities. It is hard to see a principled objection to these or, in Kantian terms, a maxim governing withholding one's information other than to protect one's informational privacy whilst enjoying the benefits of others' contributions. So the

FRA works for standard public health activities. Second, it is nonetheless true that public health can involve activities to which there might be principled – political, philosophical, religious and so on – objections. So the FRA for a duty to contribute health data has to be hedged. A simple example is the proviso on a duty to contribute one's data that it will never be used for commercial gain by private sector institutions. How many other provisos are required needs further analysis, but the FRA for a duty to contribute health data can be shored up by stipulation – personal information will only be further used for standard public health objectives, or not for commercial gain, and so on – until it becomes implausible that withholding one's data is principled in the way vaccine dissension might well be.

EXTENT OF THE DUTY

In the discussion so far, Ballantyne and Schaefer's argument has been adapted and augmented to endorse a duty to contribute personal health data for public health purposes. Now we need to get into the details as to the sorts of personal data to which this duty applies. Ballantyne and Schaefer (2018: 292) 'define health information as health and biological data derived from medical records, genome sequences, biomarkers, body and brain scans, data from clinical trials or observational studies, and lifestyle information collected directly by individuals'. This is a very expansive definition which includes various sorts of data that introduce disparate ethical and governance issues. For example, people might well agree to a duty to allow access to one's electronic medical records, whilst being much more concerned about their genetic information; the mention of clinic trials seems to take us back to the sort of invasive 'interventional research' which belongs in the original discussion of a duty to participate in biomedical research; and 'lifestyle information collected directly by individuals' takes us beyond health data routinely collected in the health care system. So, endorsing a duty to contribute personal health data for public health requires a further discussion as to quite what sorts of information this duty applies.

There is space here for some suggestions and a strategic framework. The strength of a duty to contribute depends on the sort of data in question. Specifically, the more the arguments presented in this chapter apply to data, the stronger the obligation to allow access. To recall those arguments: the negative argument was that objections to a general duty to participate in research do not apply to public health data; the positive argument was the FRA for a duty to contribute information for further public health uses. So, a paradigm is that there is a strong duty to allow access to one's electronic medical records (EMRs) for further use in support of standard public health activities. The negative argument works well here: none of the arguments against an obligation to participate in biomedical research, such as unequal distribution of benefits and violations of bodily integrity, apply. And the positive argument works well too: to enjoy the public health benefits that accrue from further uses of other people's EMRs whilst withholding one's own is free riding. In turn, and given the caveat discussed in the previous section (such as, no commercial gain, for example), consent is not required.

How far to go from this paradigm requires more detailed analysis, but in the strategic framework suggested here, there are two key questions. What dissimilarities exist between the paradigm and the case under discussion? And are those dissimilarities ethically relevant? To illustrate, contrast EMRs with biobanked samples and novel forms of personal health information such as social media data. Regarding the former, there are two obvious dissimilarities between personal information in EMRs versus biobanks: collecting biological samples require bodily invasion, and they carry genetic information. But are these ethically salient?

One could argue that the latter is more relevant than the former. After all, enormous quantities of biological samples are routinely collected in a health system for standard diagnostic and treatment purposes. Typically this requires consent, and is fully justified by the interests of patients. But once acquired, such materials seem much like any other store of personal health information, including EMRs; as such, the argument for a duty to contribute them for public health purposes would apply. But the genetic information carried in biological samples is a serious (and much discussed) consideration, because the data are not personal to just the individual whose material it is, but to genetically related others. Since this is an ethically relevant dissimilarity, different regulatory mechanisms, and even different consent requirements, might apply.

The same schema applies to novel forms of personal health information such as social media data. The question is whether social media data can be treated like EMRs, in that there is a duty to contribute and so there is no consent requirement on its further use for public health purposes. And, again, the key is whether there are ethically relevant dissimilarities between these. For example, one might say that EMRs are quite different to social media data, because the former is of direct relevance to health care, whereas the vast majority of social media data are not at all directly heath related. But is this dissimilarity ethically salient?

Take, for example, the 'lifestyle information' mentioned by Ballantyne and Schaefer: social media is full of information about health-related behaviour, choices, trends and lifestyles that would be invaluable in public health; why does it matter that the data were not originally directly health related? But other dissimilarities seem ethically very relevant. An obvious example recalls the fact that public health is a state sanctioned endeavour. To allow the intrusion by the state into one's social media profile for the sake of public health is antithetical to liberal assumptions about state intrusion into the private sphere.

CONCLUDING REMARKS

To summarise the response recommended in this chapter to the consent problem in public health, the overall strategy is to 'divide and conquer'. Four categories of public health data were distinguished by reference to the consent requirement. The first category does not raise a consent problem for public health over and above that which arises in the ongoing critique of the 'individual voluntary informed consent' paradigm. The second comprises data collection that does not require consent. There is a consent requirement on the third category of data, but it can be outweighed. This distilled public health's consent problem down to the hard case of secondary uses of personal data. A two-part argument for a duty to provide one's health information for further uses in support of public health was presented. The negative part trades on Ballantyne and Schaefer's suggestion that the main objections to a duty to participate in medical research do not apply to health data research. The positive part is a free riding argument for a duty to contribute personal data for public health. How far this duty extends requires further analysis. An important caveat is that there is no duty to provide one's data for purposes to which one has a principled objection. And the sources of health information – EMRs, biobanks, social media, for example – to which the duty to contribute one's data applies requires further analysis.

Chapter 7

Trust and Trustworthiness

This book aims to defend public health information from unnecessarily restrictive policies. But privacy concerns are heightened by a 'crisis of trust', including in institutions responsible for public health data. Building trust in public health data management by improving regulation goes a long way towards addressing this. But better regulation needs bolstering because it cannot be the sole strategy. The suggestion pursued here starts with a striking difference in how trust is discussed in public health as opposed to philosophical literature. Philosophical analysis distinguishes the interpersonal attitude of trust from cognate attitudes, such as confidence, a distinction which is not made in the public health discussion. Eliding this distinction obscures a research question: might trust, as it figures in philosophical analyses, help bolster the confidence-building regulatory changes called for by public health advocates?

This seems unpromising, because philosophers think of trust as an interpersonal attitude, whereas public trust is required in public health. But Townley and Garfield (2013) have argued for public trust, in the philosophical sense, in professionals and institutions. Their view is defended and applied to trust in institutions responsible for public health information. The upshot is that there are two ways to reassure the public about how their information is used for public health purposes. First, improved regulatory mechanisms ensure reliability and build confidence (as recommended in the public health literature). Second, the fundamental principles and values of public health institutions ensure their trustworthiness, which encourages and justifies public trust (of the sort that figures in the philosophical literature). This strategy is defended and its application is discussed.

TRUST, PUBLIC HEALTH AND PRIVACY

Trust has been a recurrent issue throughout the history of public health and the briefer history of public health ethics. One reason is that public health requires government involvement and state intrusion into individual lives for the good of the community and – at least in liberal political cultures – there is widespread mistrust of government (a point to which we return later in this discussion). This was recognised in early public health ethics literature: 'To succeed, the field of public health must gain the public's trust that the inevitable higher proportions of government involvement and population targeting imposed by public health, relative to other branches of health care, are appropriate' (Kass 2001: 1782).

As the discipline of public health ethics continued to develop from around the turn of the century, seminal texts referred to trust. One persistent theme was that a sound ethics of public health is required in order to generate trust. Callahan and Jennings (2002: 172), for example, recommended 'building up a body of ethical principles and standards that would protect the trust and legitimacy the [public health] profession should maintain'. Another trust-related theme in public health ethics is that interventions should be evaluated by reference to trust. A recent example is Wilkinson's (2017: 264) insightful discussion of countermanipulation in public health, which argues that 'loss of trust is likely to be a compelling objection to counter-manipulation in some cases but not all cases'.

More specifically, trust is central to the problematic addressed in this book, namely, the privacy-utility dilemma in the context of public health information. The overall aim is to defend public health data from overly restrictive policies motivated by increased concerns about privacy. Trust has an inverse relationship with privacy concerns. The less people trust institutions responsible for public health data, the greater their privacy concerns; the more people trust institutions responsible for public health data, the less their privacy concerns. In turn, levels of trust determine willingness to contribute information (electronic health records, biological samples and so on) for public health purposes; in particular, mistrust reduces willingness to contribute, which inevitably results in lost utility.

So, high levels of trust in institutions responsible for managing public health data is clearly conducive to the aim in this book of protecting public health information. What makes this so challenging is the oft-reported crisis of trust in public institutions. It is very common to read that levels of trust in institutions ranging from governments to health care systems to professionals is low and getting lower. If this is true – and assuming it includes institutions responsible for managing public health information – the prospect is bleak:

given the inverse relation just mentioned, the upshot is heightened privacy concerns, unwillingness on the part of a sceptical public to contribute data, increased demand for strict regulation and lost public health benefits.

BUILDING TRUST

But things are not so bleak. For one thing, building trust is a prominent theme in recent literature on public health information. For example, Lee and Gostin (2009) recognised that 'Public health agencies . . . collect, store, and use personal health and behavior data to meet their legal obligation to identify and control health threats or evaluate and improve public health programs or services', suggesting that the 'foundation for this collection of health data is public trust'. They go on to propose a 'national strategy for protecting public health data', comprising ten 'ethical guidelines for the collection, storage, and use of public health data', ranging from specific requirements (such as security measures to protect records) to more general obligations (responsible stewardship, for example). Explicitly, according to Lee and Gostin, their proposal 'will safeguard not only data, but also the public's trust in the nation's public health enterprise'.

The structure of Lee and Gostin's thinking – enhanced regulatory measures and mechanisms to build public trust in public health data management – is repeated innumerable times in the public health literature. For example, McGraw et al. (2009) propose: 'Building privacy and security protections into health information technology systems will bolster trust in such systems and promote their adoption'; so they present 'a comprehensive framework that implements core privacy principles, adopts trusted network design characteristics, and establishes oversight and accountability mechanisms'. These include specific measures, such as tightening up on allowing secondary use of personal data for marketing and – interestingly, in light of the previous chapter – tougher consent rules, which could include special consent for research uses of data. In the UK, the Nuffield Council on Bioethics (2015) repeatedly stressed that regulatory mechanisms and other responses to the challenge of using health data are crucial to ensuring trust and avoiding distrust: 'Unless there are trustworthy governance systems in place that can engage with and reflect reasonable expectations in continuously evolving circumstances, initiatives that could have wide public benefits may continue to be challenged' (S.6.69; see also Larson 2013).

The same theme is applied to specific sorts of public health data. For example, Rynning (2007) points out that 'electronic health records (EHRs) can make possible immediate, even automatic transfer of patient data [including] for quality assurance, disease surveillance, public health monitoring and research', and explicitly states that the 'success of EHR systems will depend on public trust in their compatibility with fundamental rights, such as privacy and confidentiality'. Moodley and Singh (2016), focusing on biobanking in South Africa, suggest: 'Building trust will best be achieved via a system of governance structures and processes that precede the establishment of a biobank and monitor progress'. Childress and Bernheim (2008) look at emergency preparedness, including 'collection of population data during a disease outbreak' advocating that 'a primary goal should be the development and maintenance of relationships of trust'.

We could go on – other work targets data which cross-cut the themes reported above, such as McGraw's (2013) public trust approach to de-identified data, and Anderson and Edwards's (2010) work on trust and secondary data analysis – but the point is clear. The public health literature is full of references to building public trust in information management, including plausible and effective changes to regulatory mechanisms to achieve this. This forms a crucial part of the argument in this chapter. The sorts of regulatory changes repeatedly called for and described in the public health literature are fully supported here. Improving regulatory measures can engender public trust which, in turn, would alleviate the privacy concerns which motivate an unwillingness to contribute information and overly restrictive data management policies.

LIMITATIONS

But this cannot be the sole strategy. For one thing, there is an obvious irony in addressing overregulation of public health information by further regulation. Of course, the idea is to build trust by improving, not simply increasing, regulation. But in practice it is hard to do the former without the latter, because the most eye-catching way of building trust is to publicise more, as opposed to better, regulations; conversely, it is much harder to engender trust by persuading the public that less regulation is better because it is more sophisticated or precisely targeted or whatever. Hence, calls to build trust tend to result in regulation inflation.

Building trust by regulation alone would be unsatisfactory for other reasons. For one thing, improved regulation tends to shift rather than resolve the trust problem, because even if the public approve of a new regulatory measure, they may still mistrust institutions and professionals responsible for its implementation. This phenomenon has long been recognised and was perfectly captured in Power's (1994) classic analysis of one sort of regulatory mechanism, i.e. audit: 'Rather than solving the problem of trust [new forms of audit] displace it . . . there is a regress of mistrust in which the performances of auditors and inspectors are themselves subject to audit' (p. 13). This problem persists; for example, in his most recent critique of external regulation of health and social care providers, Sheldon (2019) comments: 'No system of external measurement and regulation will be able to substitute for the relations of trust and professionalism that can help promote quality'.

Another worry – particularly acute in the current context – is that regulation cannot envision and counter all possible data misuses. This creates a dilemma, because regulatory mechanisms need to be very broad in order to cover a wide array of breaches, but are then too vague to deal adequately with specific violations. And even if, at any one time, a regulatory mechanism was perfectly attuned to current informational risks, there would be a further problem, because information technology is developing so rapidly and unpredictably that regulators are always playing catch-up, so the public inevitably remain anxious about regulating for unforeseen data violations. There was a clear example of this in the discussion of anonymity and reidentification science in chapter 5: the main argument against reliance on anonymity in public health information management is not that reidentification science is currently powerful, but that we can infer from striking reidentification success that it will continue apace and in unanticipated ways.

ANALYSES OF TRUST

The upshot of the discussion so far is that regulatory changes to provide reassurance to a sceptical public are crucial to protecting public health information, but these need augmenting with further strategies. The suggestion pursued here starts with the fact that, so far in this discussion, and throughout the public heath literature, 'trust' is taken as read and used in the familiar and everyday sense. But trust is the subject of detailed analyses in various disciplines. This raises a research question: Might some insights from analyses of trust be relevant to public health information? Specifically, might such insights help to augment the strategy of 'building trust' by improving regulatory mechanisms governing public health data?

The Philosophical Analysis of Trust

In pursuing this we have to be selective, because trust is the subject of a massive literature, including quite different disciplinary and theoretical perspectives, and little consensus. So here we focus on the philosophical analysis of trust – later in this discussion, sociological critiques of trust and organisations are important – and home in on one well-established and relatively uncontroversial distinction.

The philosophical analysis of trust starts with the striking variety of goals in life which we only achieve by depending on other people (McLeod 2015). Important and intimate relationships – with spouses and partners, family members, friends – are based on mutual dependence. Our doxastic lives depend on the testimony of others – when asking someone for directions, for example – which is why trust is an epistemological issue. And we can only solve many of our practical problems – getting the car fixed and so on – by depending on people with the relevant expertise. In all such cases, one lacks certainty; for example, there is no guarantee that one's partner is faithful, an interlocutor is telling the truth or a car mechanic is going to do a good job. So dependency is risky, and one is unavoidably vulnerable in these interactions to the depended-upon party (Becker 1996).

The relevant insight in the philosophical literature is that different interpersonal attitudes – i.e. the attitude one person adopts towards another – are in play in the sorts of interactions just described. The interpersonal attitude towards one's spouse or best friend is different to that adopted in everyday circumstances, such as asking someone for directions or handing over the car to a mechanic. Typically, this difference is captured in the philosophical literature by distinguishing trust from confidence or reliance: we trust our spouse or partner or best friend; we have confidence in, or rely on, someone we ask for directions or a car mechanic (Baier 1986). Correlatively, in the philosophical literature, the property which elicits our trust is trustworthiness – we trust our best friend because we judge him or her to be trustworthy – whereas our confidence is gained when the trusted party evinces reliability (I was confident enough to give my car to that garage because I think it is reliable).

Some further details will help clarify the distinction. A standard way of establishing the difference between trust and confidence appeals to the phenomenology of being let down. Trusting makes one vulnerable to betrayal, whereas misplaced confidence creates only disappointment (cf. O'Neil 2012). To find out one's partner is having an affair, for example, is to experience the deepest feelings of hurt, loss, anger and so on, which would be quite inappropriate to having been mischievously misdirected by a stranger or fleeced by a garage. One suggested reason for this is a difference in what motivates the depended-upon party. Trust is appropriate when the trusted party will act for the sake of the trustor – i.e. because of awareness of, and concern for, their vulnerability and well-being – and to maintain the relationship. This grounds the trusted party's trustworthiness (Jones 2012). By contrast, confidence can be gained in all sorts of other ways: social pressure (to tell the truth), rewards and punishments (getting paid and stroppy customers) and so on. Hence, placing confidence is characterised by a calculative judgement as to how reliable others are, which would be out of place in trusting relations.

Trust, Confidence and Public Health Data

This philosophical distinction between trust and confidence does not figure in the public heath literature. For example, in their calls to 'build trust' in institutions responsible for public health information, public health commentators use terms such as 'trust' and 'confidence' interchangeably. To give a few from innumerable examples, the Nuffield Council on Bioethics (2015) calls for '*trustworthy* governance systems' in order to 'secure public *confidence*' (S.6.69). Kim et al. (2017) suggest that the more robust technology infrastructure required by learning health care systems 'relies on the *trust* and *confidence* of individuals'. One of Ballantyne and Schaefer's (2018) worries about enforcing the obligation to contribute health data for research (discussed in the previous chapter) is that it 'could significantly undermine public *trust* in researchers as well as health systems [and result in] lack of *confidence* in researchers' respect for their rights and autonomy'. Eliding the distinction between trust and confidence is particularly striking in works to which trust is central. For example, Resnik's (2018) book on research ethics is oriented around trust, but he eschews 'technical or esoteric' definitions – his citations make clear he has the philosophical literature in mind (p. 88) – in order to follow 'common usage of the word found in dictionaries', so he defines *trust* in terms of '*reliance* or *dependence*' (Resnik 2018: 88; cf. O'Neill 2002: 12-16). (All emphases in this paragraph added.)

Trust and trustworthiness are distinguished from confidence, reliance and reliability in the philosophical, but not the public health, literature. In one sense, this is unimportant. As a merely terminological issue it is easily sorted out. When public health commentators call for regulatory changes to institutions responsible for managing information, as reported previously – for example, Lee and Gostin's 'national strategy for protecting public health data', or McGraw et al.'s (2009) proposal to build 'privacy and security protections into health information technology systems' – they elide the philosophical distinction between trust and confidence. So, from a philosophical point of view, such regulatory changes will not build 'trust' – this is an interpersonal attitude reserved for intimate relations, such as between spouses and best friends – but, rather, will reassure the public that institutions are reliable, and thereby gain their confidence. There is nothing more substantive than terminology at issue here (for an interesting linguistic analysis, focused on public attitudes toward the police, see Cao 2015).

But in another sense, it does matter. To recall, regulatory changes to encourage the public to contribute their information for public health is a crucial but limited strategy, so we were looking to bolster it. Eliding the distinction between trust and confidence obscures an important possibility. Might trust of the kind that figures in the philosophical analysis – i.e. trust and trustworthiness, as opposed to (mere) confidence or reliance and reliability – be relevant to the relationship between the public and institutions responsible for public health information? Could calls for regulatory changes be augmented by building trust in the sense in which philosophers understand that term?

This might seem hopeless. As outlined above, trust in the philosophical sense refers to an interpersonal attitude appropriate only in very intimate personal relationships, which are quite different to the relationship between the public and institutions responsible for their health information. So, to apply trust in the philosophical sense to the public's relationship to institutions would seem to be a category error. But there is longstanding interest in institutional trust (Govier 1997), the trust-reliance distinction is drawn in discussions of attitudes towards organisations (Cohen and Dienhart 2013), and the distinction informs a sizeable literature on trust in health care systems (Zhao et al. 2019) and between health care professionals and their patients (Ozawa and Sripad 2013). So the idea that there might be public trust in institutions, analogous to the interpersonal trust philosophers identify, survives initial scepticism.

PUBLIC TRUST

To pursue this, it will be useful to focus closely on an advocate. Townley and Garfield (2013) argue that the philosophical understanding of trust applies to institutions and professionals. They start with the philosophical 'distinction between trust and reliance' – in making the contrast with trust, they tend to use 'reliance' as opposed to 'confidence' – recognising that it is usually thought of as 'a distinction between kinds of interpersonal relations'; but, they claim, 'trust is not only an interpersonal matter', because we 'individually or collectively trust, distrust, rely on, or fail or refuse to rely on . . . institutions or institutional players' (p. 95).

Their dialectical strategy is to illustrate how both trust and reliance are required in our relationships to professionals and institutions, respectively, by reference to the academy. So, first, they describe university teachers who are trustworthy but unreliable, or reliable but untrustworthy; then they show how a university is an institution that 'could fail in terms of reliability or in terms of trust'. They end by acknowledging the limits of public trust, describing the sorts of institutions, and relations to them, which determine whether public trust or mere reliance is warranted, again by reference to universities.

Public Trust and Betrayal

How plausible is Townley and Garfield's suggestion? One worry is that important aspects of the philosophical analysis of trust do not seem appropriate to 'public trust'. For example, betrayal is a key feature of the philosophical analysis: someone who places his or her trust is vulnerable to betrayal, whereas misplaced confidence results in mere disappointment. So, Townley and Garfield's claim that we trust (as well as rely on) professionals and institutions entails that we are vulnerable to betrayal (not mere disappointment) by professionals and institutions. Hence they say: 'Trust and its betrayal, as well as reliance and its disappointment, are not restricted to the private sphere. They have public dimensions as well'; and they go on to 'shed light on the structure and value of public trust and the dangers of betrayal of such trust', by reference to the academy, i.e. university teachers who betray their student's trust, and universities which betray the public's trust (p. 97).

Is this really plausible, especially in light of certain features of betrayal? The difference between betrayal and disappointment is not the magnitude of seriousness. Some betrayals of trust are relatively minor – it ended what turned out to be an unimportant relationship – whereas disappointment can be very serious (confidence in an unreliable garage will get you killed). The difference is phenomenological: the felt experience of betrayal is very different to that of disappointment. Is it really feasible that an institution could elicit such feelings? Relatedly, as Townley and Garfield are aware,

> The goods of trust and the harms of betrayal, unlike the goods and harms pertaining to reliance, are not fungible. A failure of mere reliability can be offset by a compensatory or symmetrical benefit. . . . If trust has been breached, however, it makes no sense to compensate (p. 97).

But whilst this is surely true of interpersonal betrayal – a relationship is irreparably damaged by an affair, for example – is it really plausible of institutions? Surely it always at least 'makes sense' to require an institution to compensate for their unreliability.

Species of Trust

In responding to these sorts of worries, a suggestion by Holland and Stocks (2017) is helpful. So far, the discussion in this chapter has retained the traditional distinction between trust and confidence (or reliance). But Holland and Stocks present a tripartite analysis in which there are three relevant interpersonal attitudes. First, confidence (or reliance) is as it figures in the traditional distinction. But Holland and Stocks then distinguish two species of trust, which they call specific trust and general trust. Akin to reliance, specific trust is an attitude one person (A) adopts toward another (B) in order to achieve a goal (X); but the relationship between A and B has developed in ways that make it more than mere reliance (Hardin 2002). Holland and Stocks illustrate this by contrasting the mere reliance one places in a taxi service, with the example of a passenger who comes to know his or her regular taxi driver over a period of time, and thereby starts to trust the driver (in the 'specific' sense) to get him or her to places on time. Holland and Stocks reserve 'general trust' for a second species of trust, one that figures in the kinds of very intimate relationships, such as between spouses and partners, best friends and so on, described here.

The important point for present purposes is that betrayal is a defining feature of the three attitudes Holland and Stocks distinguish. As in the traditional distinction, what they mean by confidence (or reliance) threatens only disappointment, not betrayal. But betrayal figures differently in the two species of trust. Regarding general trust, they say: 'Betrayal here is profound and shocking, causing intense psychological harm; the harm penetrates all the deeper because trust at this stratum is stripped bare of any of the psychological defences present in other interpersonal attitudes' (p. 271). By contrast, this sort of devastation is not threatened by specific trust. For example, if the taxi driver the passenger trusts in the 'specific' sense fails to get him or her to a place on time, it would be inappropriate for the passenger to feel there had been a 'profound and shocking betrayal' or 'intense psychological harm', and hyperbolic to suggest there had.

Holland and Stocks's suggestion can help to defend Townley and Garfield's 'public trust' argument from the objection that professionals and institutions cannot really betray us. The objection commits a category error. It is certainly questionable whether professionals and institutions can cause betrayal that is 'profound or shocking', or 'intense psychological harm'. But that is only an objection to 'public trust' on the assumption that our attitude to professionals and institutions is one of 'general trust'. In fact, in Holland and Stocks's terms, the sort of trust the public has in professionals and institutions is one of 'specific trust'. Typically, a relationship between a person and a professional or an institution develops which grounds an attitude that is more than mere reliance, but not full-on general trust. Since this does not threaten betrayal of the sort that occurs in intimate relationships, the objection that such betrayal is implausible founders.

Trust and Professionals

Townley and Garfield's 'public trust' is plausible; furthermore, specific objections to their presentation do not apply in the present context. One example homes in on Townley and Garfield's discussion of public trust in professionals (as opposed to institutions). They describe Terry the teacher, who is trustworthy but unreliable. For example, her student, Lia, 'might become exasperated with Terry's unreliability [yet] still properly regard her as trustworthy' (p. 98). Evidently, this example works if and only if the very same individual is both unreliable and trustworthy (otherwise, it would be like saying, I trust my wife but rely on my car mechanic). Technically speaking, the referents of 'Terry' and 'her' in the previous quote must be numerically identical. But Terry has a dual identity, being both a person and a professional. The worry is that Terry could be trustworthy *qua* person, but unreliable *qua* teacher. In which case, the referents of 'Terry' and 'her' are numerically nonidentical, so there is no evidence here that the trust-reliance distinction applies to professionals.

This objection is difficult to meet because we often distinguish between people *qua* person and professional. We often say things like, 'I don't like him as person, but he's a damn good dentist' or 'I'm not going back to that butcher, but I'll miss his sense of humour'. Similarly, it is common to see the professional 'mask' slip to reveal the person, or for someone to switch from being a friendly person to an austere professional. To echo Townley and Garfield's illustration, all university teachers have experienced relating to students in these different modes – more as persons than professionals, or vice versa – for example, when a supervision session becomes less academic and pastoral care is required, or a joking relation has to be curbed because the student has failed to hand in an assignment.

But although this is a difficult objection, it is specific to the sort of professional relationship epitomised by Townley and Garfield's illustration of teachers and their students. These are clearly one-to-one relationships and admit of interactions ranging from the purely professional to the more personal. Hence, it was easy to suggest that Lia relates to Terry *qua* person versus *qua* professional. But when we adapt their argument to public trust and public health information, this problem just falls away. Obviously, both professionals and institutions are relevant to public health data, because institutions responsible for managing public health information are run by professionals. But members of the public do not relate to public health officials in anything like the way students and teachers relate to one another. Terry and Lia, for example, have a one-to-one relationship, and there is no equivalent to that in public health, because individual members of the public do not relate on a one-to-one basis with individual public health professionals. So we can leave this objection to Townley and Garfield moot, because, though it applies to their example, it is irrelevant to the present argument about public trust in public health institutions.

PUBLIC TRUST AND PUBLIC HEALTH INSTITUTIONS

Public trust – i.e. the view that trust, and not only confidence or reliance, extends to the public's relationship to professionals and institutions – is defensible. But there are lots of different sorts of institutions to which the public relates in various ways. Whether trust is relevant, and how trust interplays with confidence or reliance, will depend on the institution in question. So the next issue is whether public trust is relevant in the specific case of institutions responsible for managing public health data.

Townley and Garfield (2013: 103ff.) acknowledge this issue, saying that there 'are public institutions of different kinds to which the public as a whole or individual members of a society bear very different kinds of relations'. Reliance, trust and the interplay between these will vary from institution to institution, and 'there are no general rules governing where each is appropriate'. Townley and Garfield discuss this in terms of what they call 'the limits of trust'. Staying with academic illustrations, they contrast two sorts of higher education institutions – 'Sophist College' and 'Generic University'– in order to tease out the role of trust and its interplay with reliance or confidence.

Here there is a dialectical oddity, because Townley and Garfield's discussion tends to focus on institutionalised relationships – between students and teachers, or colleagues, or teachers and their employers – whereas the important question is when the public's relationship to whole institutions (as opposed to individual or small groups of professionals) is one of trust and not just reliance. Still, the important suggestion Townley and Garfield make is that the relevance of public trust to an institution depends on values:

> Public institutions that are the repositories and beneficiaries of public trust make tacit or explicit commitments to uphold certain values. . . . Many such values cannot thrive without such interdependent institutions and without these institutions enjoying public trust. This entails that these institutions are proper objects of moral reactive attitudes as well as parties to contracts, with attendant obligations for compensation when they fail to perform reliably in their purely instrumental roles (p. 103).

Trust and Shared Values

That trust and trustworthiness in some way depend on shared values is well established (Lahno 2001). The basic idea that trust is warranted by value congruence between the trustor and trusted parties informs sociological critiques of trust and confidence in institutions and organisations.

An informative example is Tonkiss and Passey's (1999) classic study of trust and confidence in UK voluntary sector organisations, including informal voluntary associations and 'third sector' institutions, such as charities. Their analysis was based on the now-familiar 'distinction between *trust* – as pertaining to ethical relations which are not conditioned by an external framework of controls – and *confidence* – referring to relations which are secured by contract or other regulatory forms, and which proceed on the basis of rational expectations' (p. 258). Tonkiss and Passey's 'theoretical discussion suggested that trust is closely linked to values, and issues of trust in relation to voluntary organisations rest heavily on public identification with the values these organisations represent' (p. 264). So, sociological critique of trust in organisations supports Townley and Garfield's suggestion that public trust is elicited by values: the public trusts – as opposed to merely being confident of, or relying on – institutions and organisations when it recognises and shares their core values.

This gives us a handle on whether public trust is relevant to institutions responsible for managing public health information: do they 'make tacit or explicit commitments to uphold certain values' of the sort that elicit public trust? It would seem so, because there is a good deal of value congruence here. The core values of public health – population health, communal benefit, the importance of protecting the most vulnerable and so on – are shared by most thoughtful and well-meaning members of the public. Hence, it is unsurprising when Tonkiss and Passey (1999: 261–262) report empirical evidence that, although people 'trust charities "a great deal" or "mostly" to be honest and fair', they trust health related institutions, 'including the National Health Service', even more. For all that this is old data – and the NHS is not focussed on managing public health information – such findings resonate because they are explained by the theoretical connection between trust and values: the public trust (not merely rely on) public health institutions, because it recognises and shares their core values.

In sum, the strategy advocated in this chapter is this. Trust is crucial to protecting public health information. And trust in institutions is said to be low. This can be met by regulatory changes to institutions managing public health data, made in order to gain public confidence (as opposed to trust), as called for in the public health literature. These are crucial, but insufficient. So we should augment these by also gaining public trust (as opposed to confidence). This is feasible because the general notion of public trust is theoretically defensible, and it is promising because of the value congruence between the public and institutions responsible for managing public health data.

CHALLENGES

Before going on to the practical application of this line of thought, some objections need to be addressed. One refers back to Tonkiss and Passey (1999). The main argument in their paper is that changes in the environment of the British voluntary sector was causing a shift in its basis from trust to confidence: 'greater regulation, competition, professional fundraising, corporate sponsorship and a "contract culture" means that voluntary organisations are increasingly governed by mechanisms designed to develop and maintain confidence . . . [which] potentially undercut its resources of trust' (p. 272). In other words, confidence and trust are mutually exclusive. This is clearly inimical to the strategy of augmenting regulatory changes to public health data management, which are designed to build confidence, by also gaining public trust: if regulatory changes to build public confidence 'undercut trust', the strategy is hopeless.

To meet this challenge, we can appeal to salient differences between sorts of institutions. Organisations of the sort studied by sociologists – such as charities in the British voluntary sector analysed by Tonkiss and Passey – create a confidence-trust dilemma by starting to look more and more like businesses. For example, when a charity employs corporate means to raise funds, or when a number of similar charities start competing with one another for donations in the way businesses do, people stop trusting them. The basis of this is that people are distrustful of profit-oriented businesses with strong corporate identities; in other words, value congruence is replaced by value dissonance. Institutions managing public health information differ in two main respects.

First, they are not after the public's money – at least, they ought not to be (we will return to this later) – so there is no prospect of becoming increasingly financially avaricious. Second, they are not competing with one another for a market share, so there is no prospect of becoming adversarial in the way familiar in corporate culture. In terms borrowed from the preceding quote, we can endorse 'greater regulation' of institutions responsible for public health data, without worrying that this 'undercuts trust', because none of the other changes to the operating environment, such as 'competition, professional fundraising . . . etc.' are relevant. So, public health is well placed to meet the challenge that greater regulation and fostering trust are mutually exclusive.

Mistrust of Government

There is a stronger challenge to the suggestion that the public might trust, and not merely rely on, public health institutions responsible for their data. Public health institutions are agents of the state and as has long been recognised, and mentioned at the start of this chapter, the public are distrustful of governments and their agencies. This challenge to public trust in public health institutions is not easily met.

For example, the obvious response is to appeal to the 'democratic mandate': at least in developed democracies, public trust in government agencies is warranted by the political legitimacy ensured by democratic processes. So the public need not mistrust public health institutions *qua* government agents, because the public has endorsed the government and its agencies. But this is bound to be unsatisfactory. Mistrust of government is prevalent in democracies, so appealing to the democratic mandate clearly does not work. And it is easy to see why. Generally, in complex, developed democracies, individuals are too far removed from political decision making to feel reassured that they can trust government agents (Holland 2009). And specific attempts to enhance democratic legitimation – opinion polls, citizens' juries and so on – fall well short of providing the requisite reassurance to engender public trust (O'Neill 2002: 170–174).

A better way to meet this challenge is to ask how forceful it is in the specific case of public trust in institutions responsible for managing public health information. What really elicits public mistrust toward state-backed public health? People are particularly suspicious of state coercion, i.e. being forced by the state to act against their will in the name of public health. This is most obvious in cases of paternalistic public health policies, i.e. interventions which coerce people for their own good (for example, by enforcing healthy or removing unhealthy options). Paternalistic policies elicit familiar complaints about the 'nanny state', which are colloquial expressions of liberal concerns about state intrusion into the private sphere and the basis of public disquiet about state-backed public health.

But this has little to do with public health information *per se*. Of course there is an indirect connection, because paternalistic public health policies are evidence based. But the vast majority of public health work – and associated information management – is not of the sort that elicits public distrust because it is state sanctioned. Preventive measures (such as screening programmes and mass immunization), public health surveillance and monitoring systems, responses to public health emergencies, and so on do not create public distrust, based on general mistrust of government. It is only when the public feels that public health has gone too far – in particular, in being objectionably paternalistic – that the involvement of government elicits public distrust. So we can fully acknowledge the well-established fact that the public mistrust governments and their agents – and even that the public has serious misgivings about the role of the state in public health interventions which flout individual liberty or autonomy – whilst promoting public trust in public health information management.

APPLICATION

To recap, public health literature advocates regulatory improvements to build public trust in data collection and management. Philosophers distinguish trust and trustworthiness from confidence and reliability. So, in philosophical terms, public health advocates are encouraging public confidence (not trust) in information management. This raises the possibility that trust and trustworthiness – as understood in philosophy – and not only confidence and reliability, are relevant to public health data management. In turn, this suggests two ways of reassuring the public about the handling of public health information: regulatory changes of the sort recommended in the public health literature to build public confidence in public health data management, and fostering public trust in institutions responsible for public health information, based on shared core values.

Public health institutions are well placed to complement building confidence, as suggested in the public health literature, with fostering public trust, as suggested here. The public do not think of public health and its constituent professionals and organisations in the way they do a secondhand car dealership or a bank, i.e. fundamentally untrustworthy institutions on which they are obliged, more or less resentfully and suspiciously, to rely. Public health should trade on this public perception of trustworthiness by taking every opportunity to reiterate the public health values shared by the public and, conversely, distancing public health from activities which undermine public trust. As Alfano and Huijts (forthcoming) put it, in a different context, 'corporations and institutions have strong instrumental and moral reasons to adopt a suite of policies that promote their appearing trustworthy and being trustworthy'.

Commercialism is a good illustration. To recall, the challenge posed by Tonkiss and Passey (1999) discussed in the previous section is that building confidence and gaining trust are mutually exclusive. This was said to apply to some institutions, such as avaricious commercial organisations, but not to public health. For example, public health, unlike the commercial sector, is not after people's money. But commercialisation is a long-established and persistent worry about some sorts of public health activities, including those involving information, such as public concern about the (mis)use of a UK biobank for commercial purposes (Levitt and Weldon 2005). So, in order to foster public trust by retaining and communicating values shared by the public – and distancing itself from the wrong values (ones that undermine public trust) – it is crucial that public health institutions explicitly disavow using health information for commercial purposes.

The basic idea is that value congruence exists and should be protected and fostered. One specific way to do this refers to a subtheme in the public health literature, namely, elicitation studies to reveal ‘determinants of trust’. (In light of the foregoing discussion, ‘trust’ in the following quotes is what philosophers mean by ‘confidence’ or ‘reliance’.) Devising regulatory changes to reassure the public is helped by knowing what predisposes people to share or withhold their data, and what works in shifting their predisposition from withholding to sharing. This generates analyses of determinants of individuals’ preparedness to share health information, and their preferences for specific sorts of regulatory mechanisms.

For example, Dinev et al. (2016) argue for the importance of understanding ‘individuals’ attitudes regarding EHR [electronic health records] and the factors that influence them’, finding that ‘perceived effectiveness of regulatory mechanisms positively impact trust’ (p. 19). Kim et al.’s (2017) study of ‘factors that affect consumers’ willingness to share electronic health information for healthcare and research’ found that individuals’ choices were influenced by ‘attitudes toward EHRs as well as beliefs about research benefit and individual control’. Bansal, Zahedi and Gefen (2010) took a similar approach to the willingness of online users to disclose health information, revealing the ‘intrinsic factors (individuals’ dispositions) that impact online trust’ (p. 139).

Given the argument of this chapter, we need an equivalent research agenda for trust and trustworthiness, as opposed to confidence and reliability. In other words, we need empirically informed analyses of public trust in institutions responsible for public health data. There are suitable models. For example, Kehoe and Ponting’s (2003) analysis of determinants of public trust is based on just the sort of value congruence presented here, but it is focused on health care reform; we need equivalent sorts of empirical analyses for information management. As an initial suggestion, this can mirror the established subtheme of ‘determinants of trust’ just referred to: what predisposes individuals to trust or mistrust public health institutions? And what works in terms of shifting their predisposition from an attitude of mistrust to trust? More specifically, given that public trust is grounded in shared values, the empirical focus must be on values. What is the public’s understanding of the values espoused by public health institutions? Which values ground the public’s perception of public health institutions as trustworthy? What can institutions responsible for managing public health information do to foster or lose the public’s trust? So this chapter can be read as conceptual groundwork for empirical analysis of people’s predisposition to trust, and not merely rely on, public health institutions.

TRUST, TRUSTWORTHINESS AND DEFENDING PUBLIC HEALTH INFORMATION

As a coda to this chapter, it is worth highlighting how the strategy of augmenting public confidence with public trust bolsters arguments in defence of public health information presented in preceding chapters. For example, the problematic that developed in chapters 2 and 3 was overregulation, i.e. bringing all public health practice under the purview of governance would be impracticable and undesirable. This difficulty was met by proportionate review and ethical screening. But proportionality could be viewed suspiciously by a public with heightened privacy concerns, because it could be seen as a risky reduction in oversight of personal data. Persuading the public that they should remain confident because this is better, not less, regulation is extremely difficult; so trust is crucial, because the more the public feels that institutions managing their data are trustworthy, the less they will be concerned by systems of proportionality, such as ethical triage.

Likewise, on the basis of the dualist account of privacy defended in chapter 4, chapter 5 argued for reliance on anonymity in data governance despite the threat of reidentification. But this could well be viewed suspiciously by a public with privacy concerns, to whom it might seem disingenuous to retain the binary anonymous-identifiable model given the rise of reidentification science. We could try to retain or regain the public's confidence by improving de-identification techniques and analysing reidentification risks. But this will only get us so far, and public trust is crucial here. For example, the argument in chapter 5 turned on the unlikelihood of public health data being reidentified, and the more the public think institutions responsible for managing public health data are trustworthy, the less concerned they will be that those institutions will reidentify their data, or will expose their data to reidentification risks by external adversaries.

Chapter 6 appealed to Mill's harm principle to justify public health information. Once again, this might be viewed suspiciously by a distrustful public. For example, as discussed, the principle can be interpreted so widely as to justify any government intrusion, on the grounds that some sort of risk of third-party harm is thereby avoided. This is part of the challenge discussed earlier in this chapter that public health institutions are agents of government, and it is extremely hard to regulate against. So once again, trust is crucial. The more a sceptical public can trust public health institutions because they think of them as trustworthy, the less anxious they will be about unjustifiable state incursions into their informational privacy on grounds of third-party harms.

A final example: the previous chapter argued that consent is not as big a problem in public health data management as might appear. Lots of public health information does not create serious consent problems, and genuine hard cases, particularly regarding secondary use of personal data, were countered by an argument for a duty to provide information for public health purposes. But consent is a principal mechanism by which people control access to and use of their information, so any dilution of the right to consent might well be viewed suspiciously. Again, regulation is part of the answer – co-opted data for public health purposes had better be well regulated – but trust is crucial, because the more people think of public health institutions responsible for their data as trustworthy, the less concerned they will be by weakening the consent requirement.

CONCLUDING REMARKS

A dialectical pattern has clearly emerged. Preceding discussions in this book focused on important underlying features of public health information: governance, privacy, anonymity, harms and consent, respectively. Each discussion culminated in an argument in favour of public health information. But a sceptical public with heightened privacy concerns might find all this suspicious. In each case, building confidence by regulation is important. But this has to be augmented by fostering public trust: the more people think of the institutions responsible for managing their data as trustworthy, the more their suspicions will be alleviated.

Conclusion

As mentioned at the end of the Introduction, each of the preceding chapters can be read independently as a substantive discussion, but there is an overarching argument. This was quickly summarised in the Introduction and has been alluded to at various points in the text, but we can now set out the argument more fully. The overall aim of the book is to defend public health information from overly restrictive data regulation and management. Why is this necessary, and how does the book achieve it?

DATA PROTECTION AND PUBLIC HEALTH INFORMATION

To see why public health information needs defending requires putting the utility-privacy dilemma in the context of the 'information (or digital) age'. There is unprecedented and increasing capacity for generating, acquiring, linking and sharing personal data. This includes increasingly powerful information technologies, seemingly ubiquitous social media and ever larger data sets. Generally speaking – and not to focus on public health in particular – this information revolution deepens the utility-privacy dilemma, because both social utility and privacy concerns are commensurate with the amount of personal data generated. In other words, the more personal data that is produced, the greater are the potential social benefits and people's informational privacy concerns.

But the information revolution has not just deepened the dilemma, because there is also a discernible general tendency to prioritise privacy protection over social utility. This is entirely understandable. The sheer amount and variety of personal data generated, and the potential for serious misuse, are bound to heighten informational privacy concerns. Also, not all personal data have social utility; much of it is created by individuals for their own convenience – commercial, social, entertainment and so on – and not to any great social purpose. In this case, the social utility falls away, but the privacy concerns remain. So it is unsurprising that, of the two parts of the dilemma, privacy protection tends to be prioritised over social utility.

The inevitable result is increasingly restrictive data regulation and management. A ready example at the time of writing this is the European Union's General Data Protection Regulation (GDPR), which came into force in 2018. The GDPR tightens restrictions on how personal data can be acquired and used and imposes requirements on information-gathering institutions, such as publicising their legal basis for holding personal information, whilst increasing penalties for noncompliance. This is a Eurocentric example of a worldwide phenomenon: over 80 countries currently have privacy laws of some sort in place. The general trend for all such data regulation is towards increasing privacy protection in the form of more stringent data regulation and management.

Data regulation tends not only towards the more restrictive, it also tends towards the indiscriminate, in that it applies to a wide variety of sorts of information. The GDPR is again illustrative, because it imposes restrictions on 'personal data [which] means *any information* relating to an identified or identifiable natural person' (emphasis added). There are always caveats – for example, around what is meant by 'sensitive data' and so on – but the general point is that data regulation tends to have wide coverage of information of quite different sorts. In this respect it is useful to talk domains of information – such as financial and commercial, security related, health related, consumer information and so on – the point being that privacy legislation tends to apply to information in many such domains.

But restrictive data legislation is not equally appropriate to all domains of information. This is because the utility-privacy dilemma plays out differently in different domains. For example, personal financial information promises relatively little social utility but comparatively high privacy risks. So restrictive data protection legislation and increased privacy protection are entirely appropriate to that domain of information. But by contrast, public health information promises very great social utility and comparatively low privacy risks. So those same restrictive data legislation and management policies are less appropriate here.

To reemphasis a point made a number of times in the main text, this is not to downplay the deep privacy concerns, including serious informational risks and harms, which public health information can occasionally create.

Nonetheless, public health has got caught up in a general response to heightened privacy concerns and increased informational risks generated in the information age. The upshot is increasingly restrictive regulation and management of public health data, to the detriment of public health and, in turn, society in general.

DEFENDING PUBLIC HEALTH INFORMATION

The book's general strategy in response is to analyse and evaluate two things: first, the privacy concerns and informational risks associated with public health; second, the resources available for meeting them. In brief, the overall argument is that the former are overstated whilst the latter are understated. Each part of this strategy can be illustrated in turn by pulling together some of the themes in the preceding discussions.

Public health is frequently said to raise 'privacy concerns'. But what does that actually mean? In light of the extended discussion of privacy in chapter 3, such claims are ambiguous between privacy *qua* personal space and informational control. The former is deeply significant, but the latter is germane to public health. So, the failure in the public health literature to disambiguate 'privacy concerns' tends towards overstatement. Associating public health data with 'privacy' is bound to ring loud alarm bells, because everyone is very concerned about his or her privacy. But concerns are muted by pointing out that privacy *qua* personal space is largely irrelevant. Hence, analysing privacy reveals and corrects for an overstatement of public health's privacy problem.

Likewise, it is frequently stated that public health data generate serious risks and harms. The analysis of privacy shows that the privacy concerns relevant to public health are consequentialist; i.e. there are risks of very harmful disclosures of public health information. There is no denying here that these can be serious. But how serious, and in what ways? The discussion in chapter 5 suggests that the risks and harms associated with public health information are systematically overstated. Commentators tend to hand wave by gesturing towards standard cases – stigmatisation, HIV status, mental illness – which creates the false impression that all public health data are (as in these particular cases) highly dangerous. And there are subtler forms of overstatement, such as associating public health informational privacy with one's conception of the good, as analysed in chapter 5.

So there is a tendency to overstate the privacy concerns and informational risks associated with public health. Conversely, the resources available to manage these are understated. For one thing, we can and should continue to rely on anonymisation in public health. This is crucial, because whole swathes of public health data can be anonymised, and it would be a governance disaster to mistrust anonymisation. The challenge to this, as discussed in chapter 4, is reidentification. But striking reidentifications of data give the false impression that powerful adversaries are intent on reidentifying everything. This is another source of overstatement: exaggerating the threat of reidentification overstates public health informational concerns. In fact, the risk of reidentification of specifically public health data is low, and can (and should) be lowered. Of course this is not without its risks, but so is failure to rely on anonymisation, because unnecessary data restrictions compromise public health.

The main text emphasises other underused resources to defend public health information. Mill's harm principle, discussed in chapter 5, is a case in point. The principle is vexed; but its noncontentious core is that some impositions are justified on grounds of third-party harms, and this clearly applies to a good deal of standard public health information gathering. Likewise, the discussion of consent in chapter 6. There is another source of overstatement here, as commentators frequently reiterate how impracticable it is to gain consent in public health; in fact, as explained in chapter 6, the consent problem in public health distils down to further uses of extant data. The underused resource proposed for dealing with this is the duty to provide public health information. This duty should be more rigorously defended and required in public health. Finally, as argued in chapter 7, public trust is an underused resource for defending public health information. Appeals to build confidence by making regulatory changes to make institutions more reliable are already established; but these can be augmented by gaining the public's trust in trustworthy institutions which share their core values.

References

Alfano, Mark, and Nicole Huijts. Forthcoming. 'Trust and Distrust in Institutions and Governance.' Forthcoming in *The Routledge Handbook of Trust and Philosophy,* edited by Judith Simon. Routledge.

Allhoff, Fritz. 2005. 'Free-Riding and Research Ethics.' *The American Journal of Bioethics* 5, no. 1: 50–51.

Al-Saggaf, Yeslam, and Md Zahidul Islam. 2015. 'Data Mining and Privacy of Social Network Sites' Users: Implications of the Data Mining Problem.' *Science and Engineering Ethics* 21, no. 4: 941–966.

Al-Shahi, Rustam, and Charles Warlow. 2000. 'Using Patient-Identifiable Data for Observational Research and Audit: Overprotection Could Damage the Public Interest.' *British Medical Journal* 321: 1031–1032.

Altman, Irwin. 1977. 'Privacy Regulation: Culturally Universal or Culturally Specific?' *Journal of Social Issues* 33, no. 3: 66–84.

Anderson, Nick, and Kelly Edwards. 'Building a Chain of Trust: Using Policy and Practice to Enhance Trustworthy Clinical Data Discovery and Sharing.' In *Proceedings of the 2010 Workshop on Governance of Technology, Information and Policies*. ISBN: 978-1-4503-0446-7.

Angst, Corey M. 2009. 'Protect my Privacy or Support the Common-good? Ethical Questions about Electronic Health Information Exchanges.' *Journal of Business Ethics* 90, supplement 2: 169–178.

Baier, Annette. 1986. 'Trust and Antitrust.' *Ethics* 96, no. 2: 231–260.

Baily, Mary Ann, Melissa M. Bottrell, Joanne Lynn and Bruce Jennings. 2006. 'Special Report: The Ethics of Using QI Methods to Improve Health Care Quality and Safety.' *Hastings Center Report* 36, no. 4: S1–S40.

Ballantyne, Angela, and G. Owen Schaefer. 2018. 'Consent and the Ethical Duty to Participate in Health Data Research.' *Journal of Medical Ethics* 44, no. 6: 392–396.

Bambery, Ben, Michael Selgelid, Charles Weijer, Julian Savulescu and Andrew J. Pollard. 2015. Ethical Criteria for Human Challenge Studies in Infectious Diseases.' *Public Health Ethics* 9, no. 1: 92–103.

Bansal, Gaurav, Fatemeh 'Mariam' Zahedi and David Gefen. 2010. 'The Impact of Personal Dispositions on Information Sensitivity, Privacy Concern and Trust in Disclosing Health Information Online.' *Decision Support Systems* 49, no. 2: 138–150.

Bayer, Ronald, and Amy L. Fairchild. 2004. 'The Genesis of Public Health Ethics.' *Bioethics* 18, no. 6: 473–492.

Bean, Sally, Blair Henry, J. Michelle Kinsey, Keitha McMurray, Catherine Parry and Tiffany Tassopoulos. 2010. 'Enhancing Research Ethics Decision-Making: An REB Decision Bank.' *IRB: Ethics & Human Research* 32, no. 6: 9–12.

Bean, Sally. 2010. 'Beyond Research Exceptionalism: A Call for Process Redesign.' *The American Journal of Bioethics* 10, no. 8: 58–60.

Beauchamp, Tom L., and Yashar Saghai. 2012. 'The Historical Foundations of the Research-Practice Distinction in Bioethics.' *Theoretical Medicine and Bioethics* 33, no. 1: 45–56.

Becker, Lawrence C. 1996. 'Trust as Noncognitive Security about Motives.' *Ethics* 107, no. 1: 43–61.

Benitez, Kathleen, and Bradley Malin. 2010. 'Evaluating Re-Identification Risks with Respect to the HIPAA Privacy Rule.' *Journal of the American Medical Informatics Association* 17, no. 2: 169–177.

Bernheim, Ruth Gaare, James F. Childress, Alan Melnick and Richard J. Bonnie. 2013. *Essentials of Public Health Ethics*. Burlington MA: Jones & Bartlett Publishers.

Biletzki, Anat, and Anat Matar. 2018. 'Ludwig Wittgenstein.' In *The Stanford Encyclopedia of Philosophy* (Summer 2018 edition), edited by Edward N. Zalta. https://plato.stanford.edu/archives/sum2018/entries/wittgenstein/

Black, Nick. 2003. 'Secondary Use of Personal Data for Health and Health Services Research: Why Identifiable Data are Essential.' *Journal of Health Services Research & Policy* 8, supplement 1: 36–40.

Bloustein, Edward J. 1964. 'Privacy as an Aspect of Human Dignity: An Answer to Dean Prosser.' *New York University Law Review* 39, no. 6: 962–1007.

Bortolotti, Lisa, and Bert Heinrichs. 2007. 'Delimiting the Concept of Research: An Ethical Perspective.' *Theoretical Medicine and Bioethics* 28, no. 3: 157–179.

Boslaugh, Sarah. 2007. *Secondary Data Sources for Public Health: A Practical Guide*. Cambridge University Press.

Bradley, Ben. 2012. 'Doing Away with Harm.' *Philosophy and Phenomenological Research* 85, no. 2: 390–412.

Brakewood, Beth, and Russell A. Poldrack. 2013. 'The Ethics of Secondary Data Analysis: Considering the Application of Belmont Principles to the Sharing of Neuroimaging Data.' *Neuroimage* 82: 671–676.

Brand, Angela, Tobias Schulte and Nicole M. Probst-Hensch. 2012. 'Biobanking for Public Health.' In *Trust in Biobanking*, edited by Peter Dabrock, Jochen Taupitz, and Jens Ried, 3–20. Berlin: Springer.

Brassington, Iain. 2007. 'John Harris' Argument for a Duty to Research.' *Bioethics* 21, no. 3: 160–168.

Brassington, Iain. 2014. 'The Case for a Duty to Research: Not Yet Proven.' *Journal of Medical Ethics* 40, no. 5: 329–330.

Brochhausen, Mathias, Jie Zheng, David Birtwell, Heather Williams, Anna Maria Masci, Helena Judge Ellis and Christian J. Stoeckert. 2016. 'OBIB – A Novel Ontology for Biobanking.' *Journal of Biomedical Semantics* 7, no. 1: 23.

Buchanan, David R., and Franklin G. Miller. 2006. 'A Public Health Perspective on Research Ethics.' *Journal of Medical Ethics* 32, no. 12: 729–733.

Budin-Ljøsne, Isabelle, Harriet Teare, Jane Kaye and Deborah Mascalzoni. 2015. 'Meta Consent: Is it New and Is It Fit for Purpose?' *British Medical Journal* 350: h2146.

Burke, Wylie, Hilary Burton, Alison E. Hall, Mohamed Karmali, Muin J. Khoury, Bartha Knoppers, Eric M. Meslin, et al. 2010. 'Extending the Reach of Public Health Genomics: What Should Be the Agenda for Public Health in an Era of Genome-Based and "Personalized" Medicine?' *Genetics in Medicine* 12, no. 12: 785–791.

Burris, Scott, James Buehler and Zita Lazzarini. 2003. Applying the Common Rule to Public Health Agencies: Questions and Tentative Answers about a Separate Regulatory Regime. *The Journal of Law, Medicine & Ethics* 31, no. 4: 638–653.

Callahan, Daniel, and Bruce Jennings. 2002. 'Ethics and Public Health: Forging a Strong Relationship.' *American Journal of Public Health* 92, no. 2: 169–176.

Calo, Ryan. 2011. 'The Boundaries of Privacy Harm.' *Indiana Law Journal* 86, no. 3: 1131–1162.

Campbell, Lori D., Jonas J. Astrin, Yvonne DeSouza, Judith Giri, Ashokkumar A. Patel, Melissa Rawley-Payne, Amanda Rush et al. 2018. 'The 2018 Revision of the ISBER Best Practices: Summary of Changes and the Editorial Team's Development Process.' *Biopreservation and Biobanking* 16, no. 1: 3–6.

Candib, Lucy M. 2007. 'How Turning a QI Project into Research Almost Sank a Great Program.' *The Hastings Center Report* 37, no. 1: 26–30.

Cao, Liqun. 2015. 'Differentiating Confidence in the Police, Trust in the Police, and Satisfaction with the Police.' *Policing: An International Journal of Police Strategies & Management* 38, no. 2: 239–249.

Caplan, Arthur L. 'Is There a Duty to Serve as a Subject in Biomedical Research?' *IRB: Ethics & Human Research* 6, no. 5: 1–5.

Cave, Emma, and Christopher Nichols. 2007. 'Clinical Audit and Reform of the UK Research Ethics Review System.' *Theoretical Medicine and Bioethics* 28, no. 3: 181–203.

Cavoukian, Ann, and Khaled El Emam. 2011. *Dispelling the Myths Surrounding De-Identification: Anonymization Remains a Strong Tool for Protecting Privacy.* Information and Privacy Commissioner of Ontario, Canada. http://www.ontla.on.ca/library/repository/mon/25006/310614.pdf

Cavoukian, Ann, and Daniel Castro. 2014. 'Big Data and Innovation, Setting the Record Straight: De-Identification *Does* Work.' Office of the Information and Privacy Commissioner, Onatario, Canada. Available at, http://www2.itif.org/2014-big-data-deidentification.pdf

CDC. 2010. 'Distinguishing Public Health Research and Public Health Nonresearch.' Centers for Disease Control and Prevention, Office of the Associate Director for Science. Available at, https://www.cdc.gov/od/science/integrity/docs/cdc-policy-distinguishing-public-health-research-nonresearch.pdf

Chalmers, Don, Dianne Nicol, Jane Kaye, Jessica Bell, Alastair V. Campbell, Calvin W. L. Ho, Kazuto Kato, et al. 2016. 'Has the Biobank Bubble Burst? Withstanding the Challenges for Sustainable Biobanking in the Digital Era.' *BMC Medical Ethics* 17: 39.

Chalmers, Iain. 2007. 'Regulation of Therapeutic Research is Compromising the Interests of Patients.' *International Journal of Pharmaceutical Medicine* 21, no. 6: 395–404.

Chan, Sarah, and John Harris. 2009. 'Free Riders and Pious Sons – Why Science Research Remains Obligatory.' *Bioethics* 23, no. 3: 161–171.

Chen, Lu-Yen A., and Tonks N. Fawcett. 2017. 'Service Evaluation: A Grey Area of Research?' *Nursing Ethics*. https://doi.org/10.1177/0969733017742961

Childress, J. 2013: 'Surveillance and Public Health Data: The Foundation and Eyes of Public Health'. In *Essentials of Public Health Ethics*, edited by Ruth Gaare Bernheim, James F. Childress, Alan Melnick and Richard J. Bonnie, 97–118. Burlington MA: Jones & Bartlett Publishers.

Childress, James F., and R. Gaare Bernheim. 2008. 'Public Health Ethics.' *Bundesgesundheitsblatt-Gesundheitsforschung-Gesundheitsschutz* 51, no. 2: 158–163.

CIOMS. 2009. *International Ethical Guidelines for Epidemiological Studies*. Council for International Organizations of Medical Sciences (CIOMS). Geneva, Switzerland: WHO Press, ISBN: 92-9036-081-X.

Clarke, Roger. 2006. 'What's 'Privacy'?' *Australian Law Reform Commission Workshop*. http://www.rogerclarke.com/DV/Privacy.html

Cline, Jay. 2009. 'Privacy Matters: When Is Personal Data Truly De-Identified?' *Computerworld*, July 24, 2009.

Code of Federal Regulations. Part 46: Protection of Human Subjects. Available at, http://www.gpo.gov/fdsys/pkg/CFR-2007-title45-vol1/pdf/CFR-2007-title45-vol1-part46.pdf.

Cohen, Marc A., and John Dienhart. 2013. 'Moral and Amoral Conceptions of Trust, with an Application in Organizational Ethics.' *Journal of Business Ethics* 112, no. 1: 1–13.

Coleman, Michel P., Barry G. Evans and Geraldine Barrett. 2003. 'Confidentiality and the Public Interest in Medical Research – Will We Ever Get it Right?' *Clinical Medicine* 3, no. 3: 219–228.

Conway, Mike. 2014. 'Ethical Issues in Using Twitter for Public Health Surveillance and Research: Developing a Taxonomy of Ethical Concepts from the Research Literature.' *Journal of Medical Internet Research* 16, no. 12: e290.

Créquit, Perrine, Ghizlène Mansouri, Mehdi Benchoufi, Alexandre Vivot and Philippe Ravaud. 2018. 'Mapping of Crowdsourcing in Health: Systematic Review.' *Journal of Medical Internet Research* 20, no. 5: e187.

Cullity, Garrett. 1995. 'Moral Free Riding.' *Philosophy & Public Affairs* 24, no. 1: 3–34.

Culnane, Chris, Benjamin I. P. Rubinstein and Vanessa Teague. 2017. 'Health Data in an Open World.' *arXiv preprint: 1712.05627.*

Dare, Tim. 1998. 'Mass Immunisation Programmes: Some Philosophical Issues.' *Bioethics* 12, no. 2: 125–149.

Davies, Hugh, F. Wells, and M. Czarkowski. 2009. 'Standards for Research Ethics Committees: Purpose, Problems and the Possibilities of Other Approaches.' *Journal of Medical Ethics* 35, no. 6: 382–383.

De Souza, Yvonne G., and John S. Greenspan. 2013. 'Biobanking Past, Present and Future: Responsibilities and Benefits.' *AIDS* 27, no. 3: 303–312.

Debatin, Bernhard. 2011. 'Ethics, Privacy, and Self-Restraint in Social Networking.' In *Privacy Online*, edited by Sabine Trepte and Leonard Reinecke, 47–60. Berlin: Springer.

DeCew, Judith. 2018. 'Privacy.' In *The Stanford Encyclopedia of Philosophy* (Spring 2018 Edition), edited by Edward N. Zalta. https://plato.stanford.edu/archives/spr2018/entries/Privacy/

Department of Health. 2005. *Report of the Ad Hoc Advisory Group on the Operation of NHS Research Ethics Committees.* Available at, https://webarchive.nationalarchives.gov.uk/20130124070050/http://www.dh.gov.uk/prod_consum_dh/groups/dh_digitalassets/@dh/@en/documents/digitalasset/dh_4112417.pdf

Dinev, Tamara, Valentina Albano, Heng Xu, Alessandro D'Atri and Paul Hart. 2016. 'Individuals' Attitudes Towards Electronic Health Records: A Privacy Calculus Perspective.' In *Advances in Healthcare Informatics and Analytics*, edited by Gupta Ashish, Vimla L. Patel, and Robert A. Greenes, 19–50. Cham: Springer.

Dowd, Michael. 2010. 'Contextualised Concerns: The Online Privacy Attitudes of Young Adults.' In *Privacy and Identity Management for Life,* edited by Simone Fischer-Hübner, Penny Duquenoy, Marit Hansen, Ronald Leenes and Ge Zhang, 78–89. Dordrecht: Springer.

Dunkel, Yaron F. 2001. 'Medical Privacy Rights in Anonymous Data: Discussion of Rights in the United Kingdom and the United States in Light of the Source Informatics Cases.' *Loyola of Los Angeles International and Comparative Law Review* 23, no. 1: 41–79.

Edwards, S. J. L., and R. Omar. 2008. 'Ethics Review of Research: In Pursuit of Proportionality.' *Journal of Medical Ethics* 34, no. 7: 568–572.

El Emam, Khaled, Elizabeth Jonker, Luk Arbuckle and Bradley Malin. 2011. 'A systematic Review of Re-Identification Attacks on Health Data.' *PLOS ONE* 6, no. 12: e28071.

El Emam, Khaled, Sam Rodgers and Bradley Malin. 2015. 'Anonymising and Sharing Individual Patient Data.' *British Medical Journal* 350: h1139.

El Emam, Khaled. 2010. 'Risk-Based De-Identification of Health Data.' *IEEE Security & Privacy* 8, no. 3: 64–67.

Engle, Eric. 2012. 'The History of the General Principle of Proportionality: An Overview.' *Dartmouth Law Journal* 10, no. 1: 1–23.

Eriksson, Stefan, and Gert Helgesson. 2005. 'Potential Harms, Anonymization, and the Right to Withdraw Consent to Biobank Research.' *European Journal of Human Genetics* 13, no. 9: 1071.

Faden, Ruth R., Nancy E. Kass, Steven N. Goodman, Peter Pronovost, Sean Tunis and Tom L. Beauchamp. 2013. 'An Ethics Framework for a Learning Health Care System: A Departure from Traditional Research Ethics and Clinical Ethics.' *Hastings Center Report* 43, supplement 1: S16–S27.

Fairchild, Amy L., and Ronald Bayer. 2004. 'Ethics and the Conduct of Public Health Surveillance.' *Science* 303, no. 5658: 631–632.

Fairchild, Amy L., and Ronald Bayer. 2016. 'In the Name of Population Well-Being: The Case for Public Health Surveillance.' *Journal of Health Politics, Policy and Law* 41, no. 1: 119–128.

Finn, Rachel L., David Wright and Michael Friedewald. 2013. 'Seven Types of Privacy.' In *European Data Protection: Coming of Age*, edited by Serge Gutwirth, Ronald Leenes, Paul De Hert and Yves Poullet, 3–32. Dordrecht: Springer.

Forsberg, Joanna Stjernschantz, Mats G. Hansson and Stefan Eriksson. 2014. 'Why Participating in (Certain) Scientific Research Is a Moral Duty.' *Journal of Medical Ethics* 40, no. 5: 325–328.

Fransson, Martin N., Emmanuelle Rial-Sebbag, Mathias Brochhausen and Jan-Eric Litton. 2015. 'Toward a Common Language for Biobanking.' *European Journal of Human Genetics* 23, no. 1: 22–28.

Freund, Paul A. 1971. 'Privacy: One Concept or Many.' In *Privacy and Personality*, edited by J. Roland Pennock and John W. Chapman, 182–198. New Brunswick, NJ: Aldine Transaction.

Fritz, Fleur, Binyam Tilahun, and Martin Dugas. 2015. 'Success Criteria for Electronic Medical Record Implementations in Low-Resource Settings: A Systematic Review.' *Journal of the American Medical Informatics Association* 22, no. 2: 479–488.

Froomkin, A. Michael. 1995. 'Flood Control on the Information Ocean: Living with Anonymity, Digital Cash, and Distributed Databases.' *Journal of Law and Commerce* 15, no. 2: 395–507.

Gelinas, Luke, Alan Wertheimer and Franklin G. Miller. 2016. 'When and Why Is Research without Consent Permissible?' *Hastings Center Report* 46, no. 2: 35–43.

Gittelman, Steven, Victor Lange, Carol A. Gotway Crawford, Catherine A. Okoro, Eugene Lieb, Satvinder S. Dhingra and Elaine Trimarchi. 2015. 'A New Source of Data for Public Health Surveillance: Facebook Likes.' *Journal of Medical Internet Research* 17, no. 4: e98.

Gkoulalas-Divanis, Aris, and Grigorios Lookides (editors). 2015. *Medical Data Privacy Handbook*. Cham: Springer.

Goldberg, Daniel S. 2011. 'Eschewing Definitions of the Therapeutic Misconception: A Family Resemblance Analysis.' *Journal of Medicine and Philosophy* 36, no. 3: 296–320.

Golder, Su, Shahd Ahmed, Gill Norman and Andrew Booth. 2017. 'Attitudes Toward the Ethics of Research Using Social Media: A Systematic Review.' *Journal of Medical Internet Research* 19, no. 6: e195.

Gostin, Lawrence O. and Hodge, J. G., 2004: *Public Health Practice vs. Research: A Report for Public Health Practitioners Including Cases and Guidance for Making*

Distinctions. Council of State and Territorial Epidemiologists. Available at, http://www.cste2.org/webpdfs/CSTEPHResRptHodgeFinal.5.24.04.pdf

Gostin, Lawrence O. 1991. 'Ethical Principles for the Conduct of Human Subject Research: Population-Based Research and Ethics.' *Law, Medicine and Health Care* 19, no. 3-4: 191–201.

Gostin, Lawrence O., and Kieran G. Gostin. 2009. 'A Broader Liberty: JS Mill, Paternalism and the Public's Health.' *Public Health* 123, no. 3: 214–221.

Govier, Trudy. 1997. *Social Trust and Human Communities*. Montreal and Kingston: McGill-Queen's University Press.

Grembowski, David. 2015. *The Practice of Health Program Evaluation* (2nd edition). Thousand Oaks, CA: Sage Publications.

Gutwirth, Serge. 2002. *Privacy and the Information Age*. Translated by Raf Casert. Lanham, MD: Rowman & Littlefield Publishers.

Hanser, Matthew. 2008. 'The Metaphysics of Harm.' *Philosophy and Phenomenological Research* 77, no. 2: 421–450.

Hansson, Mats G., Hanns Lochmüller, Olaf Riess, Franz Schaefer, Michael Orth, Yaffa Rubinstein, Caron Molster et al. 2016. 'The Risk of Re-Identification Versus the Need to Identify Individuals in Rare Disease Research.' *European Journal of Human Genetics* 24, no. 11: 1553–1558.

Hansson, Sven Ove. 2011. 'Do We Need a Special Ethics for Research?' *Science and Engineering Ethics* 17, no. 1: 21–29.

Harcourt, Bernard E. 1999. 'The Collapse of the Harm Principle.' *Journal of Criminal Law & Criminology* 90, no. 1: 109–194.

Hardin, Russell. 2002. *Trust and Trustworthiness*. New York: Russell Sage Foundation.

Harman, Elizabeth. 2009. 'Harming as Causing Harm.' In *Harming Future Persons: Ethics, Genetics and the Nonidentity Problem*, edited by Melinda A. Roberts and David T. Wasserman, 137–154. Dordrecht: Springer.

Harris, John. 2005. 'Scientific Research Is a Moral Duty.' *Journal of Medical Ethics* 31, no. 4: 242–248.

Harrosh, Shlomit. 2012. 'Identifying Harms.' *Bioethics* 26, no. 9: 493–498.

Hart, Herbert Lionel Adolphus. 1955. 'Are There Any Natural Rights?' *The Philosophical Review* 64, no. 2: 175–191.

Haugaard, Mark. 2010. 'Power: A 'Family Resemblance' Concept.' *European Journal of Cultural Studies* 13, no. 4: 419–438.

Hauge, Michelle V., Mark D. Stevenson, D. Kim Rossmo and Steven C. Le Comber. 2016. 'Tagging Banksy: Using Geographic Profiling to Investigate a Modern Art Mystery.' *Journal of Spatial Science* 61, no. 1: 185–190.

Hepgul, Nilay, Katherine E. Sleeman, Alice M. Firth, Anna Johnston, James T. H. Teo, William Bernal, Richard J. B. Dobson, et al. 2019. 'In Response to Ballantyne and Schaefer's "Consent and the Ethical Duty to Participate in Health Data Research".' *Journal of Medical Ethics*. doi: 10.1136/medethics-2018-105271

Hodge Jr., James G. 2003. 'Health Information Privacy and Public Health.' *The Journal of Law, Medicine & Ethics* 31, no. 4: 663–671.

Hodge Jr., James G. 2005. 'An Enhanced Approach to Distinguishing Public Health Practice and Human Subjects Research.' *The Journal of Law, Medicine Ethics* 33, no. 1: 125–141.

Hoffman, Sharona, and Andy Podgurski. 2012. 'Balancing Privacy, Autonomy, and Scientific Needs in Electronic Health Records Research.' *Southern Methodist University Law Review* 65, no. 1: 85–144.

Holland, Stephen, and David Stocks. 2017. 'Trust and Its Role in the Medical Encounter.' *Health Care Analysis* 25, no. 3: 260–274.

Holland, Stephen. 2009. 'Public Health Paternalism – A Response to Nys.' *Public Health Ethics* 2, no. 3: 285–293.

Holland, Stephen. 2015. *Public Health Ethics* (2nd edition). Cambridge: Polity.

Holm, Søren. 2007. 'A Rose by Any Other Name... Is the Research/Non-Research Distinction Still Important and Relevant?' *Theoretical Medicine and Bioethics* 28, no. 3: 153–155.

Hunter, David, and James Wilson. 2010. 'Responses to Open Peer Commentaries on "Research Exceptionalism".' *The American Journal of Bioethics* 10, no. 8: W4–W6.

Hunter, David. 2007. 'Proportional Ethical Review and the Identification of Ethical Issues.' *Journal of Medical Ethics* 33, no. 4: 241–245.

John, Stephen. 2010. 'Three Worries about Three Arguments for Research Exceptionalism.' *The American Journal of Bioethics* 10, no. 8: 67–69.

Johnson, Ginger A., and Cecilia Vindrola-Padros. 2017. 'Rapid Qualitative Research Methods during Complex Health Emergencies: A Systematic Review of the Literature.' *Social Science & Medicine* 189: 63–75.

Joly, Yann, Stephanie O. M. Dyke, Warren A. Cheung, Mark A. Rothstein and Tomi Pastinen. 2015. 'Risk of Re-Identification of Epigenetic Methylation Data: A More Nuanced Response is Needed.' *Clinical Epigenetics* 7, no.1: Article 45.

Jonas, Hans, 1976. Philosophical Reflections on Experimenting with Human Subjects. In *Biomedical Ethics and the Law*, edited by James M. Humber and Robert F. Almeder, 217–242. Boston, MA: Springer.

Jones, Karen. 2012. 'Trustworthiness.' *Ethics* 123, no. 1: 61–85.

Kahn, Jonathan. 2002. 'Privacy as a Legal Principle of Identity Maintenance.' *Seton Hall Law Review* 33, no.1: 371–410.

Kaplan, Bonnie. 2015. 'Selling Health Data: De-Identification, Privacy, and Speech.' *Cambridge Quarterly of Healthcare Ethics* 24, no. 3: 256–271.

Karimi-Busheri, Feridoun, ed. 2015. *Biobanking in the 21st Century*. Cham: Springer.

Kasper, Debbie V.S. 2005. 'The Evolution (or Devolution) of Privacy.' *Sociological Forum* 20, no. 1: 69–92.

Kass, Nancy E. 2001. 'An Ethics Framework for Public Health.' *American Journal of Public Health* 91, no. 11: 1776–1782.

Kass, Nancy E., Ruth R. Faden, Steven N. Goodman, Peter Pronovost, Sean Tunis and Tom L. Beauchamp. 2013. 'The Research-Treatment Distinction: A Problematic Approach for Determining Which Activities Should Have Ethical Oversight.' *Hastings Center Report* 43, supplement 1: S4–S15.

Kehoe, Susan M., and J. Rick Ponting. 2003. 'Value Importance and Value Congruence as Determinants of Trust in Health Policy Actors.' *Social Science & Medicine* 57, no. 6: 1065–1075.

Kelman, Christopher W., A. John Bass and Cashel D. J. Holman. 2002. 'Research Use of Linked Health Data – A Best Practice Protocol.' *Australian and New Zealand Journal of Public Health* 26, no. 3: 251–255.

Kemeny, John G., and Paul Oppenheim. 1956. 'On Reduction.' *Philosophical Studies* 7, no. 1: 6–19.

Khoury, Muin J., and John P. A. Ioannidis. 2014. 'Big Data Meets Public Health.' *Science* 346, no. 6213: 1054–1055.

Kim, Katherine K., Pamela Sankar, Machelle D. Wilson and Sarah C. Haynes. 2017. 'Factors Affecting Willingness to Share Electronic Health Data Among California Consumers.' *BMC Medical Ethics* 18: 25.

Kim, Scott, Peter Ubel and Raymond De Vries. 2009. 'Pruning the Regulatory Tree.' *Nature* 457, no. 7229: 534–535.

Klingler, Corinna, Diego Steven Silva, Christopher Schuermann, Andreas Alois Reis, Abha Saxena and Daniel Strech. 2017. 'Ethical Issues in Public Health Surveillance: A Systematic Qualitative Review.' *BMC Public Health* 17: 295.

Klocksiem, Justin. 2012. 'A Defense of the Counterfactual Comparative Account of Harm.' *American Philosophical Quarterly* 49, no. 4: 285–300.

Kokolakis, Spyros. 2017. 'Privacy Attitudes and Privacy Behaviour: A Review of Current Research on the Privacy Paradox Phenomenon.' *Computers & Security* 64: 122–134.

Kopelman, Loretta M. 2004. 'Minimal Risk as an International Ethical Standard in Research.' *The Journal of Medicine and Philosophy* 29, no. 3: 351–378.

Korsgaard, Christine M. 1996. *Creating the Kingdom of Ends*. Cambridge University Press.

Kupfer, Joseph. 1987. 'Privacy, Autonomy, and Self-Concept.' *American Philosophical Quarterly* 24, no. 1: 81–89.

Lahno, Bernd. 2001. 'On the Emotional Character of Trust.' *Ethical Theory and Moral Practice* 4, no. 2: 171–189.

Lamb, David. 2013. *Down the Slippery Slope: Arguing in Applied Ethics*. London: Routledge.

Lane, Julia, Victoria Stodden, Stefan Bender and Helen Nissenbaum, eds. 2014. *Privacy, Big Data, and the Public Good: Frameworks for Engagement*. Cambridge University Press.

Larson, Eric B. 2013. 'Building Trust in the Power of "Big Data" Research to Serve the Public Good.' *JAMA* 309, no. 23: 2443–2444.

Lee, Lisa M. 2014. 'Health Information in the Background: Justifying Public Health Surveillance Without Patient Consent.' In *Emerging Pervasive Information and Communication Technologies (PICT)*, edited by Kenneth D. Pimple, 39–53. Dordrecht: Springer.

Lee, Lisa M., and Lawrence O. Gostin. 2009. 'Ethical Collection, Storage, and Use of Public Health Data: A Proposal for a National Privacy Protection.' *JAMA* 302, no. 1: 82–84.

Lee, Lisa M., and Stephen B. Thacker. 2011. 'Public Health Surveillance and Knowing About Health in the Context of Growing Sources of Health Data.' *American Journal of Preventive Medicine* 41, no. 6: 636–40.

Lee, Lisa M., Charles M. Heilig and Angela White. 2012. 'Ethical Justification for Conducting Public Health Surveillance without Patient Consent.' *American Journal of Public Health* 102, no. 1: 38–44.

Levine, Robert J. 1975. 'The Boundaries Between Biomedical or Behavioral Research and the Accepted and Routine Practice of Medicine.' *National Commission on the Protection of Humans Subjects of Biomedical and Behavioral Research. The Belmont Report: Ethical Principles and Guidelines for the Protection of Human Subjects of Research, Appendix* 1. DHEW Publication No. (OS) 78-0013.

Levitt, Mairi, and Sue Weldon. 2005. 'A Well Placed Trust?: Public Perceptions of the Governance of DNA Databases.' *Critical Public Health* 15, no. 4: 311–321.

Lipworth, Wendy, Paul H. Mason, Ian Kerridge and John P. A. Ioannidis. 2017. 'Ethics and Epistemology in Big Data Research.' *Journal of Bioethical Inquiry* 14, no. 4: 489–500.

López, Gustavo, Gabriela Marín and Marta Calderón. 2015. 'Characterizing Ubiquitous Systems Privacy Issues by Gender and Age.' In *Ambient Assisted Living*, edited by Ian Cleland, Luis Guerrero, and José Bravo, 247–258. Cham: Springer.

Lowrance, William. 2003. 'Learning from Experience: Privacy and the Secondary Use of Data in Health Research.' *Journal of Health Services Research & Policy* 8, supplement 1: 2–7.

Lussier, Marie-Thérèse, Claude Richard, Terri-Lyn Bennett, Tyler Williamson and Anika Nagpurkar. 2012. 'Surveillance or Research: What's In a Name?' *Canadian Family Physician* 58, no. 1: 117.

Ma, Lin, and Jaap Van Brakel. 2016. 'Revisiting Wittgenstein on Family Resemblance and Colour(s).' *Philosophical Investigations* 39, no. 3: 254–280.

Mannion, Russel, and Jeffrey Braithwaite. 2017. 'False Dawns and New Horizons in Patient Safety Research and Practice.' *International Journal of Health Policy and Management* 6, no. 12: 685–689.

Manson, Neil C. 2018. 'The Biobank Consent Debate: Why "Meta-Consent" Is Not the Solution?' *Journal of Medical Ethics*. doi: 10.1136/medethics-2018-105007.

Manson, Neil C. 2019. 'The Ethics of Biobanking: Assessing the Right to Control Problem for Broad Consent.' *Bioethics*. doi: 10.1111/bioe.12550.

Matthews, Gregory J., Ofer Harel and Robert H. Aseltine. 2016. 'Privacy Protection and Aggregate Health Data: A Review of Tabular Cell Suppression Methods (Not) Employed in Public Health Data Systems.' *Health Services and Outcomes Research Methodology* 16, no. 4: 258–270.

May, Thomas, and Ross D. Silverman. 2005. 'Free-Riding, Fairness, and the Rights of Minority Groups in Exemption from Mandatory Childhood Vaccination.' *Human Vaccines* 1, no. 1: 12–15.

McCullough, Melissa. 2010. 'One Size Does Not Fit All: The Ethical Imperative to Limit the Concept of Research Exceptionalism.' *The American Journal of Bioethics* 10, no. 8: 60–61.

McDonald, Laura, Dimitra Lambrelli, Radek Wasiak and Sreeram V. Ramagopalan. 2016. 'Real-World Data in the United Kingdom: Opportunities and Challenges.' *BMC Medicine* 14: 97.

McGinn, Colin. 2011. *Truth by Analysis: Games, Names and Philosophy*. New York: Oxford University Press.

McGrail, Kimberlyn M., Kaitlyn Gutteridge and Nancy L. Meagher. 2015. 'Building on Principles: The Case for Comprehensive, Proportionate Governance of Data Access.' In *Medical Data Privacy Handbook*, edited by Aris Gkoulalas-Divanis and Grigorios Loukides, 737–764. Cham: Springer.

McGraw, Deven, James X. Dempsey, Leslie Harris and Janlori Goldman. 2009. 'Privacy as an Enabler, Not an Impediment: Building Trust into Health Information Exchange.' *Health Affairs* 28, no. 2: 416–427.

McGraw, Deven. 2013. 'Building Public Trust in Uses of Health Insurance Portability and Accountability Act De-Identified Data.' *Journal of the American Medical Informatics Association* 20, no. 1: 29–34.

McKinnon, Andrew. 2002. 'Sociological Definitions, Language Games and the "Essence" of Religion.' *Method & Theory in the Study of Religion* 14, no. 1: 61–83.

McLeod, Carolyn. 2015. 'Trust.' In *The Stanford Encyclopedia of Philosophy* (Fall 2015 Edition), edited by Edward N. Zalta. https://plato.stanford.edu/archives/fall2015/entries/Trust/

McMahan, Jeff. 2013. 'Causing People to Exist and Saving People's Lives.' *The Journal of Ethics* 17, no. 1–2: 5–35.

McMillan, John. 2011: 'Public Health Research Ethics: Is Non-Exploitation the New Principle for Population Based Research Ethics?' In *Public Health Ethics: Key Concepts and Issues in Policy and Practice*, edited by Angus Dawson, 174–190. Cambridge University Press.

Mehlman, Maxwell J., Eric Kodish and Jessica Berg. 2018. 'Ethical Issues in the Use of Nudges to Obtain Informed Consent for Biomedical Research.' *IRB: Ethics & Human Research* 40, no. 3: 1–5.

Menzel, Paul T. 1995. 'Paper Four: Non-Compliance: Fair or Free-Riding.' *Health Care Analysis* 3, no. 2: 113–115.

Merritt, Maria W., Joanne Katz, Ramin Mojtabai and Keith P. West Jr. 2015. 'Referral of Research Participants for Ancillary Care in Community-Based Public Health Intervention Research: A Guiding Framework.' *Public Health Ethics* 9, no. 1: 104–120.

Meyer, Lukas. 2016. 'Intergenerational Justice.' In *The Stanford Encyclopedia of Philosophy* (Summer 2016 edition), edited by Edward N. Zalta. https://plato.stanford.edu/archives/sum2016/entries/justice-intergenerational/

Mikesell, Lisa, Elizabeth Bromley and Dmitry Khodyakov. 2013. 'Ethical Community-Engaged Research: A Literature Review.' *American Journal of Public Health* 103, no. 12: e7–e14.

Mill, J. S. 1989. 'On Liberty'. In *On Liberty and Other Essays*, edited by Stefan Collini. Cambridge University Press.

Mitra, Agomoni Ganguli, and Nayha Sethi. 2016. 'Conducting Research in the Context of Global Health Emergencies: Identifying Key Ethical and Governance

Issues.' Nuffield Council on Bioethics Background Paper. Available at, http://nuffieldbioethics.org/wp-content/uploads/Research-in-global-health-emergencies-background-paper.pdf.

Moodley, Keymanthri, and Shenuka Singh. 2016. '"It's all about Trust": Reflections of Researchers on the Complexity and Controversy Surrounding Biobanking in South Africa.' *BMC Medical Ethics* 17: 57.

Moore, Adam D. 2003. 'Privacy: Its Meaning and Value.' *American Philosophical Quarterly* 40, no. 3: 215–227.

Moore, Adam D. 2007. 'Toward Informational Privacy Rights.' *San Diego Law Review*. 44, no. 4: 809–845.

Moore, Adam D. 2010. 'Privacy, Public Health, and Controlling Medical Information.' *HEC Forum* 22, no. 3: 225–240.

Mourby, Miranda, Elaine Mackey, Mark Elliot, Heather Gowans, Susan E. Wallace, Jessica Bell, Hannah Smith, Stergios Aidinlis and Jane Kaye. 2018. 'Are "Pseudonymised" Data Always Personal Data? Implications of the GDPR for Administrative Data Research in the UK.' *Computer Law & Security Review* 34, no. 2: 222–233.

Muralidhara, Sachin, and Michael J. Paul. 2018. '# Healthy Selfies: Exploration of Health Topics on Instagram.' *JMIR Public Health and Surveillance* 4, no. 2: e10150.

Narayanan, Arvind, Joanna Huey and Edward W. Felten. 2016. 'A Precautionary Approach to Big Data Privacy.' In *Data Protection on the Move*, edited by Serge Gutwirth, Ronald Leenes and Paul De Hert, 357–385. Dordrecht: Springer.

Negley, Glenn. 1966. 'Philosophical Views on the Value of Privacy.' *Law & Contemporary Problems* 31: 319–325.

NHS Digital. *Hospital Episode Statistics (HES)*. Available at, https://digital.nhs.uk/data-and-information/data-tools-and-services/data-services/hospital-episode-statistics.

NHS Digital[a]. *National Data Opt-out Programme*. Available at, https://digital.nhs.uk/services/national-data-opt-out-programme.

NHS Digital[b]. Opting Out of Sharing Your Confidential Patient Information. Available at, https://mrc.ukri.org/documents/pdf/nhs-digital-and-type-2-patient-opt-outs-voct2016/.

Nsubuga, Peter, Peter Nsubuga, Mark E. White, Stephen B. Thacker, Mark A. Anderson, Stephen B. Blount, Claire V. Broome, et al. 2006. 'Public Health Surveillance: A Tool for Targeting and Monitoring Interventions.' In *Disease Control Priorities in Developing Countries* (2nd edition), edited by Dean T. Jamison, Joel G. Breman, Anthony R. Measham, George Alleyne, Mariam Claeson, David B. Evans, Prabhat Jha, et al., 997–1015. Washington (DC): World Bank and Oxford University Press.

Nuffield Council on Bioethics. 2007. *Public Health: Ethical Issues*. Available at, http://nuffieldbioethics.org/wp-content/uploads/2014/07/Public-health-ethical-issues.pdf.

Nuffield Council on Bioethics. 2015. *The Collection, Linking and Use of Data in Biomedical Research and Health Care: Ethical Issues*. Available at, http://nuffieldbioethics.org/wp-content/uploads/Biodata-a-guide-to-the-report-PDF.pdf

Ohm, Paul. 2010. 'Broken Promises of Privacy: Responding to the Surprising Failure of Anonymization.' *UCLA Law Review* 57, no. 6: 1701–1777.

Olsen, LeighAnne, Dara Aisner, and J. Michael McGinnis, eds. 2007. *The Learning Healthcare System*. Washington (DC): National Academies Press.

Ondrusek, Nancy K., Donald J. Willison, Vinita Haroun, Jennifer A. H. Bell and Catherine C. Bornbaum. 2015. 'A Risk Screening Tool for Ethical Appraisal of Evidence-Generating Initiatives.' *BMC Medical Ethics* 16: 47.

O'Neil, Collin. 2012. 'Lying, Trust, and Gratitude.' *Philosophy & Public Affairs* 40, no. 4: 301–333.

O'Neill, Onora. 2002. *Autonomy and Trust in Bioethics*. Cambridge University Press.

Östlin, Piroska, Ted Schrecker, Ritu Sadana, Josiane Bonnefoy, Lucy Gilson, Clyde Hertzman, Michael P. Kelly et al. 2011. 'Priorities for Research on Equity and Health: Towards an Equity-Focused Health Research Agenda.' *PLOS Medicine* 8, no. 11: e1001115.

Otto, Jean Lin, Mark Holodniy and Robert F. DeFraites. 2014. 'Public Health Practice is Not Research.' *American Journal of Public Health* 104, no. 4: 596–602.

Ozawa, Sachiko and Pooja Sripad. 2013. 'How do you Measure Trust in the Health system? A Systematic Review of the Literature.' *Social Science & Medicine* 91: 10–14.

Pagliari, Claudia, Don Detmer and Peter Singleton. 2007. 'Potential of Electronic Personal Health Records.' *British Medical Journal* 335: 330–333.

Pappworth, Maurice Henry. 1967. *Human Guinea Pigs: Experimentation on Man*. London: Routledge & Kegan Paul.

Paskal, Wiktor, Adriana M. Paskal, Tomasz Dębski, Maciej Gryziak and Janusz Jaworowski. 2018. 'Aspects of Modern Biobank Activity – Comprehensive Review.' *Pathology & Oncology Research* 24, no. 4: 771–785.

Paul, Michael J., and Mark Dredze. 2017. 'Social Monitoring for Public Health.' *Synthesis Lectures on Information Concepts, Retrieval, and Services* 9, no. 5: 1–183.

Petersen, Thomas Søbirk. 2014. 'Being Worse Off: But in Comparison with What? On the Baseline Problem of Harm and the Harm Principle.' *Res Publica* 20, no. 2: 199–214.

Piel, Frédéric B., Brandon L. Parkes, Hima Daby, Anna L. Hansell and Paul Elliott. 2018. 'The Challenge of Opt-Outs from NHS Data: A Small-Area Perspective.' *Journal of Public Health* 40, no. 4: e594–e600.

Platt, Jodyn, and Sharon Kardia. 'Public Trust in Health Information Sharing: Implications for Biobanking and Electronic Health Record Systems.' 2015. *Journal of Personalized Medicine* 5, no. 1: 3–21.

Ploug, Thomas, and Søren Holm. 2015a. 'Going Beyond the False Dichotomy of Broad or Specific Consent: A Meta-Perspective on Participant Choice in Research Using Human Tissue.' *The American Journal of Bioethics* 15, no. 9: 44–46.

Ploug, Thomas, and Søren Holm. 2015. 'Meta Consent: A Flexible and Autonomous Way of Obtaining Informed Consent for Secondary Research.' *British Medical Journal* 350: h2146.

Ploug, Thomas, and Søren Holm. 2016. 'Meta Consent – A Flexible Solution to the Problem of Secondary Use of Health Data.' *Bioethics* 30, no. 9: 721–732.

Ploug, Thomas, and Søren Holm. 2017. 'Eliciting Meta Consent for Future Secondary Research Use of Health Data Using a Smartphone Application – A Proof of Concept Study in the Danish Population.' *BMC Medical Ethics* 18: 51.

Ploug, Thomas, and Søren Holm. 2017a. 'Informed Consent and Registry-Based Research – The Case of the Danish Circumcision Registry.' *BMC Medical Ethics* 18: 53.

Power, Michael. 1994. *The Audit Explosion*. London: Demos.

Pronovost, Peter, Dale Needham, Sean Berenholtz, David Sinopoli, Haitao Chu, Sara Cosgrove, Bryan Sexton, et al. 2006. 'An Intervention to Decrease Catheter-Related Bloodstream Infections in the ICU.' *New England Journal of Medicine* 355, no. 26: 2725–2732.

Public Health Ontario. 2012. *A Framework for Ethical Conduct of Public Health Initiatives*. Available at, https://www.publichealthontario.ca/en/eRepository/PHO%20%20Framework%20for%20ethical%20Conduct%20of%20Public%20Health%20Initiatives%20April%202012.pdf

Rachels, James. 1975. 'Why Privacy Is Important.' *Philosophy and Public Affairs* 4, no. 4: 323–333.

Rawls, John. 1971. *A Theory of Justice*. Cambridge (MA): Harvard University Press.

Rawls, John. 1987. 'The Basic Liberties and Their Priority.' In *Liberty, Equality, and Law: Selected Tanner Lectures on Moral Philosophy*, edited by Sterling M. McMurrin, 1–87. Salt Lake City: University of Utah Press.

Resnik, David B. 2018. *The Ethics of Research with Human Subjects: Protecting People, Advancing Science, Promoting Trust*. Cham: Springer.

Rhodes, Rosamond. 2005a. 'Response to Commentators on "Rethinking Research Ethics".' *The American Journal of Bioethics* 5, no. 1: W15–W18.

Rhodes, Rosamond. 2005. 'Rethinking Research Ethics.' *The American Journal of Bioethics* 5, no. 1: 7–28.

Rhodes, Rosamond. 2017. 'When Is Participation in Research a Moral Duty?' *The Journal of Law, Medicine & Ethics* 45, no. 3: 318–326.

Rid, Annette. 2014. 'How Should We Regulate Risk in Biomedical Research? An Ethical Analysis of Recent Policy Proposals and Initiatives.' *Health Policy* 117, no. 3: 409–420.

Rivera, Suzanne M. 2014. 'Privacy v. Progress: Research Exceptionalism Is Bad Medicine.' *Health Matrix* 24: 49–64.

Rössler, Beate. 2005. *The Value of Privacy*. Translated by Rupert D. V. Glasgow. Cambridge: Polity.

Rothstein, Mark A., and Abigail B. Shoben. 2013. 'Does Consent Bias Research?' *The American Journal of Bioethics* 13, no. 4: 27–37.

Rubel, Alan. 2012. 'Justifying Public Health Surveillance: Basic Interests, Unreasonable Exercise, and Privacy.' *Kennedy Institute of Ethics Journal* 22, no. 1: 1–33.

Rueben, Matthew, Cindy M. Grimm, Frank J. Bernieri, and William D. Smart. 2017. 'A Taxonomy of Privacy Constructs for Privacy-Sensitive Robotics.' *arXiv preprint: 1701.00841*.

Rynning, Elisabeth. 2007. 'Public Trust and Privacy in Shared Electronic Health Records.' *European Journal of Health Law* 14, no. 2: 105–112.

Salloway, Mark K., Xiaodong Deng, Yilin Ning, Shih Ling Kao, Ying Chen, G. Owen Schaefer, Jacqueline Joon-Lin Chin, et al. 2016. 'A De-Identification Tool for Users in Medical Operations and Public Health.' Presented at: IEEE-EMBS International Conference on Biomedical and Health Informatics. Available at, https://ieeexplore.ieee.org/stamp/stamp.jsp?tp=&arnumber=7455951

Scanlon, Thomas. 1975. 'Thomson on Privacy.' *Philosophy & Public Affairs* 4, no. 4: 315–322.

Scanlon, Thomas. 1998. *What We Owe to Each Other*. Cambridge (MA): Harvard University Press.

Schaefer, G. Owen, Ezekiel J. Emanuel and Alan Wertheimer. 2009. 'The Obligation to Participate in Biomedical Research.' *JAMA* 302, no. 1: 67–72.

Schleidgen, Sebastian, Alma Husedzinovic, Dominik Ose, Christoph Schickhardt, Christof von Kalle and Eva C. Winkler. 2019. 'Between Minimal and Greater than Minimal Risk: How Research Participants and Oncologists Assess Data-Sharing and the Risk of Re-Identification in Genomic Research.' *Philosophy & Technology* 32, no. 1: 39–55.

Schopper, Doris, Raffaella Ravinetto, Lisa Schwartz, Eunice Kamaara, Sunita Sheel, Michael J. Segelid, Aasim Ahmad, et al. 2016. 'Research Ethics Governance in Times of Ebola.' *Public Health Ethics* 10, no. 1: 49–61.

Schröder-Bäck, Peter, and Kyriakos Martakis. 2015. 'Counterpoint: Should Childhood Vaccination Against Measles be a Mandatory Requirement for Attending School? No.' *Chest* 148, no. 4: 854–856.

Schwab, Abraham. 2010. 'The Recipe for Overreaching Regulation.' *American Journal of Bioethics* 10, no. 8: 55–56.

Schwartz, Barry. 1968. 'The Social Psychology of Privacy.' *American Journal of Sociology* 73, no. 6: 741–752.

Schwartz, Paul M., and Daniel J. Solove. 2011. 'The PII Problem: Privacy and a New Concept of Personally Identifiable Information.' *New York University Law Review* 86, no. 6: 1814–1894.

Shapshay, Sandra, and Kenneth D. Pimple. 2007. Participation in Biomedical Research Is an Imperfect Moral Duty: A Response to John Harris. *Journal of Medical Ethics* 33, no. 7: 414–417.

Sheldon, Trevor Andrew. 2019. 'Inspecting the Inspectors – Does External Review of Health Services Provide Value for Money?' *Journal of Health Services Research & Policy*. https://doi.org/10.1177/1355819619839425.

Shiffrin, Seana Valentine. 1999. 'Wrongful Life, Procreative Responsibility, and the Significance of Harm.' *Legal Theory* 5, no. 2: 117–148.

Shore, Nancy. 2006. 'Re-Conceptualizing the Belmont Report: A Community-Based Participatory Research Perspective.' *Journal of Community Practice* 14, no. 4: 5–26.

Sifunda, Sibusiso, Priscilla Reddy, Nasheen Naidoo, Shamagonam James and David Buchanan. 2013. 'Recruiting and Educating Participants for Enrollment in HIV-Vaccine Research: Ethical Implications of the Results of an Empirical Investigation.' *Public Health Ethics* 7, no. 1: 78–85.

Sinnenberg, Lauren, Alison M. Buttenheim, Kevin Padrez, Christina Mancheno, Lyle Ungar and Raina M. Merchant. 2017. 'Twitter as a Tool for Health Research: A Systematic Review.' *American Journal of Public Health* 107, no. 1: e1–e8.

Slegers, Claudia, Deborah Zion, Deborah Glass, Helen Kelsall, Lin Fritschi, Ngiare Brown and Bebe Loff. 2015. 'Why do People Participate in Epidemiological Research?' *Journal of Bioethical Inquiry* 12, no. 2: 227–237.

Sluga, Hans. 2006. 'Family Resemblance.' *Grazer Philosophische Studien* 71, no. 1: 1–21.

Snider Jr., Dixie E., and Donna F. Stroup. 1997. 'Defining Research When it Comes to Public Health.' *Public Health Reports* 112, no. 1: 29–32.

Snooks, Helen, Hayley Hutchings, Anne Seagrove, Sarah Stewart-Brown, John Williams and Ian Russell. 2012. 'Bureaucracy Stifles Medical Research in Britain: A Tale of Three Trials.' *BMC Medical Research Methodology* 12: 122.

Solove, Daniel J. 2002. 'Conceptualizing Privacy.' *California Law Review* 90, no. 4: 1087–1155.

Solove, Daniel J. 2006. 'A Taxonomy of Privacy.' *University of Pennsylvania Law Review* 154, no. 3: 477–564.

Solove, Daniel J. 2008. *Understanding Privacy*. Cambridge (MA): Harvard University press.

Souhami, Robert. 2006. 'Governance of Research that Uses Identifiable Personal Data.' *British Medical Journal* 333: 315–316.

Steel, Daniel. 2015. *Philosophy and the Precautionary Principle*. Cambridge University Press.

Stewart, Paul M., Anna Stears, Jeremy W. Tomlinson and Morris J. Brown. 2008. 'Regulation – The Real Threat to Clinical Research.' *British Medical Journal* 337: a1732.

Stewart, Richard B. 2002. 'Environmental Regulatory Decision Making Under Uncertainty.' In *An Introduction to the Law and Economics of Environmental Policy: Issues in Institutional Design*, edited by Timothy Swanson, 71–126. Bingley, UK: Emerald Group Publishing Limited.

Stockdale, Jessica, Jackie Cassell, and Elizabeth Ford. 2018. '"Giving Something Back": A Systematic Review and Ethical Enquiry into Public Views on the Use of Patient Data for Research in the United Kingdom and the Republic of Ireland.' *Wellcome Open Research* 3: 6. https://doi.org/10.12688/wellcomeopenres.13531.2

Thomson, Judith Jarvis. 1975. 'The Right to Privacy.' *Philosophy & Public Affairs* 4, no. 4: 295–314.

Tonkiss, Fran, and Andrew Passey. 1999. 'Trust, Confidence and Voluntary Organisations: Between Values and Institutions.' *Sociology* 33, no. 2: 257–274.

Townley, Cynthia, and Jay L. Garfield. 2013. 'Public Trust.' In *Trust: Analytic and Applied Perspectives*, edited by Pekka Mäkelä, and Cynthia Townley, 95–108. Amsterdam: Rodopi Press.

Tripathy, Jaya Prasad. 2013. 'Secondary Data Analysis: Ethical Issues and Challenges.' *Iranian Journal of Public Health* 42, no. 12: 1478–1479.

Tsui, Emma K., and Amy Starecheski. 2018. 'Uses of Oral History and Digital Storytelling in Public Health Research and Practice.' *Public Health* 154: 24–30.

van den Hoven, M. J. 1997. 'Privacy and the Varieties of Moral Wrong-Doing in an Information Age.' *ACM SIGCAS Computers and Society* 27, no. 3: 33–37.

Van Den Hoven, Mariette. 2012. 'Why One Should Do One's Bit: Thinking About Free Riding in the Context of Public Health Ethics.' *Public Health Ethics* 5, no. 2: 154–160.

Van Howe, Robert S., Morten Frisch, Peter W. Adler and J. Steven Svoboda. 2019. 'Circumcision Registry Promotes Precise Research and Fosters Informed Parental Decisions.' *BMC Medical Ethics* 20: 6.

van Riel, Raphael, and Robert Van Gulick. 2018. 'Scientific Reduction.' In *The Stanford Encyclopedia of Philosophy* (Summer 2018 Edition), edited by Edward N. Zalta. https://plato.stanford.edu/archives/sum2018/entries/scientific-reduction/

van Staa, Tjeerd-Pieter, Ben Goldacre, Martin Gulliford, Jackie Cassell, Munir Pirmohamed, Adel Taweel, Brendan Delaney and Liam Smeeth. 2012. 'Pragmatic Randomised Trials Using Routine Electronic Health Records: Putting Them to the Test.' *British Medical Journal* 344: e55.

Vayena, Effy, Anna Mastroianni and Jeffrey Kahn. 2012. 'Ethical Issues in Health Research with Novel Online Sources.' *American Journal of Public Health* 102, no. 12: 2225–2230.

Vayena, Effy, Marcel Salathé, Lawrence C. Madoff and John S. Brownstein. 2015. 'Ethical Challenges of Big Data in Public Health.' *PLOS Computational Biology* 11, no. 2: e1003904.

Verweij, Marcel, and Angus Dawson. 2009. 'Public Health Research Ethics: A Research Agenda.' *Public Health Ethics* 2, no. 1: 1–6.

Viens, Adrian M., and Jasper Littmann. 2015. 'Is Antimicrobial Resistance a Slowly Emerging Disaster?' *Public Health Ethics* 8, no. 3: 255–265.

Virani, Alice Hawkins, and Holly Longstaff. 2015. 'Ethical Considerations in Biobanks: How a Public Health Ethics Perspective Sheds New Light on Old Controversies.' *Journal of Genetic Counseling* 24, no. 3: 428–432.

Wade, Derick T. 2005. 'Ethics, Audit, and Research: All Shades of Grey.' *British Medical Journal* 330: 468–471.

Warlow, Charles. 2005. 'Over-Regulation of Clinical Research: A Threat to Public Health.' *Clinical Medicine* 5, no. 1: 33–38.

Warren, Samuel, and Louis Brandeis. 1890. 'The Right to Privacy.' *Harvard Law Review* 4, no. 5: 193–220.

Wazny, Kerri. 2018. 'Applications of Crowdsourcing in Health: An Overview.' *Journal of Global Health* 8, no. 1. doi: 10.7189/jogh.08.010502.

Weijer, Charles, Jeremy M. Grimshaw, Monica Taljaard, Ariella Binik, Robert Boruch, Jamie C. Brehaut, Allan Donner et al. 2011. 'Ethical Issues Posed by Cluster Randomized Trials in Health Research.' *Trials* 12: Article 100.

Wellcome Trust. 2015. *Enabling Data Linkage to Maximise the Value of Public Health Research Data.* Available at, http://eprints.uwe.ac.uk/25387/3/Data%20linkage%20final%20report.pdf

Wendler, David. 2017. 'The Ethics of Clinical Research.' In *The Stanford Encyclopedia of Philosophy* (Winter 2017 Edition), edited by Edward N. Zalta. https://plato.stanford.edu/archives/win2017/entries/clinical-research/

Wennerberg, Hjalmar. 1967. 'The Concept of Family Resemblance in Wittgenstein's Later Philosophy.' *Theoria* 33, no. 2: 107–132.

Westin, Alan F. 1967. *Privacy and Freedom*. New York: Atheneum.

WHO. *Health Topics: Public Health Surveillance*. Available at, http://www.who.int/topics/public_health_surveillance/en/.

WHO. 2017. *WHO Guidelines on Ethical Issues in Public Health Surveillance*. Available at, http://www.who.int/ethics/publications/public-health-surveillance/en/.

Wilkinson, T. Martin. 2010. 'Assessing the Case for the Regulation of Research.' *The American Journal of Bioethics* 10, no. 8: 63–65.

Wilkinson, T. Martin. 2017. 'Counter-Manipulation and Health Promotion.' *Public Health Ethics* 10, no. 3: 257–266.

Williams, Hawys, Karen Spencer, Caroline Sanders, David Lund, Edgar A. Whitley, Jane Kaye and William G. Dixon. 2015. 'Dynamic Consent: A Possible Solution to Improve Patient Confidence and Trust in How Electronic Patient Records are Used in Medical Research.' *JMIR Medical Informatics* 3, no. 1: e3. doi: 10.2196/medinform.3525.

Willison, Donald J., Nancy Ondrusek, Angus Dawson, Claudia Emerson, Lorraine E. Ferris, Raphael Saginur, Heather Sampson and Ross Upshur. 2014. 'What Makes Public Health Studies Ethical? Dissolving the Boundary Between Research and Practice.' *BMC Medical Ethics* 15: 61.

Wilson, James, and David Hunter. 2010. 'Research Exceptionalism.' *The American Journal of Bioethics* 10, no. 8: 45–54.

Wittgenstein, L. 2009. *Philosophical Investigations* (4th edition). Edited and translated by Peter Michael Stephan Hacker and Joachim Schulte. Oxford: Wiley-Blackwell.

Woollard, Fiona. 2102. 'Have We Solved the Non-Identity Problem?' *Ethical Theory and Moral Practice* 15, no. 5: 677–690.

Yentis, Steven M., and Angus Dawson. 2006. 'Medical Studies with 'No Material Ethical Issues' – An Unhelpful, Confusing and Potentially Unethical Suggestion.' *Clinical Ethics* 1, no. 4: 234–236.

Zhao, Dahai, Hongyu Zhao, and Paul D. Cleary. 2019. 'Understanding the Determinants of Public Trust in the Health Care System in China: An Analysis of a Cross-Sectional Survey.' *Journal of Health Services Research & Policy* 24, no. 1: 37–43.

Index

www.ingramcontent.com/pod-product-compliance
Ingram Content Group UK Ltd.
Pitfield, Milton Keynes, MK11 3LW, UK
UKHW041347230926
475560UK00013B/125

9 781786 600554